DOMINIC SKINNER'S
GLOWOGRAPHY

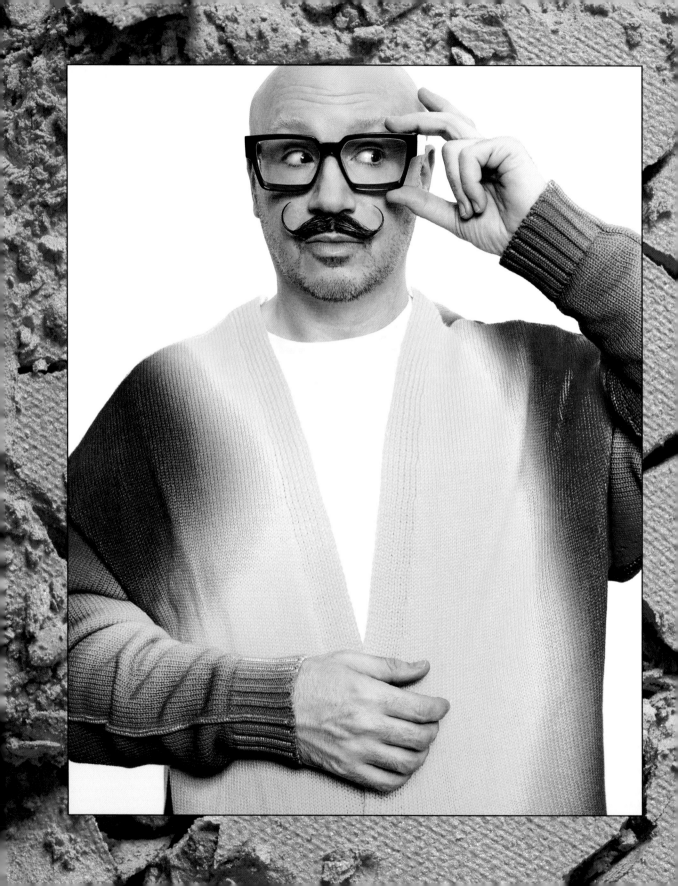

DOMINIC SKINNER'S
GLOWOGRAPHY

A PRACTICAL GUIDE
TO NEW MAKEUP

PHOTOGRAPHY BY LINDA SHAKESBY

contents

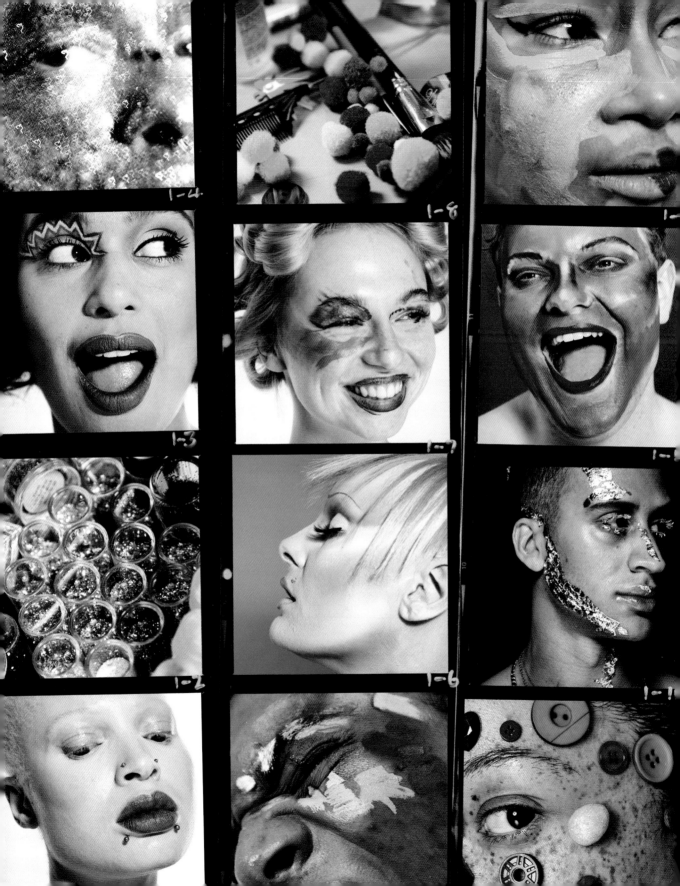

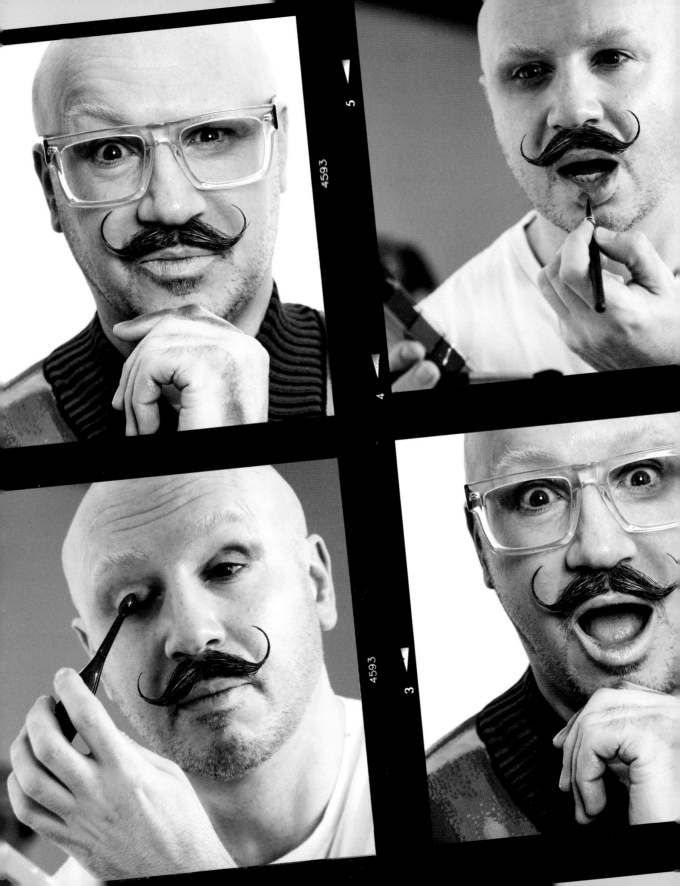

Welcome to your 'anti' how-to to makeup book

Makeup has always been on my radar, but it was never a consideration to pursue it as a career – to begin with anyway. Growing up, with two brothers who were five and seven years older, I spent a lot of time with my mum, and she loves makeup. We would walk the beauty halls of local department stores together and I would gaze happily at the shiny, well-lit displays showcasing bright colours and sleek packaging: it was like a toy shop to me. When mum needed some quiet time at home, we would play 'paint Mummy's face' – a game that consisted of her resting on the sofa with closed eyes while I used makeup brushes to stroke her face (this game abruptly ended when I decided to get creative and paint her eyelids using her latest Chanel nail enamel).

As I got older, I started to notice makeup in movies, the music world and magazines, and saw how a certain colour or style could signal your unique personality. This fostered a desire to be myself, to stand out and be seen. My curiosity about makeup was a key part of the process of establishing my own character: whether it was watching Mum go through her daily routine or witnessing Daryl Hannah spray black paint across her eyes in the movie *Blade Runner* (my gateway drug into the world of sci-fi, sparking a life-long interest in looking to the future, always striving for the next big thing).

At every stage of my life there has been a hundred different paths I could have taken, and each decision was a mix of carefully thought-out planning with both creativity and logic at its heart or just a chaotic random stumble upon. Art and reason. Both, I felt, were necessary to build something beautiful. This led me first into the world of art and design, my passion for many years until makeup returned to my life in my early twenties. Coming to makeup as a career choice later than most gave me my unorthodox take on beauty: to me, it was less about convention and more about individuality. Makeup was war paint, a flag to wave into battle, a declaration of who we are within a world of billions.

Over the years I have been asked many questions, from how to do a technique to how someone can get to do what I do. As I answered these questions I would also focus on the 'how': how, in this time of mass communication and social media are people still struggling to find the answers? What is missing from the beauty world that leaves people lost in a space that has millions of content creators and brands all screaming for you to follow them? But perhaps it's that question which gives a clue as to the answer: people are being told to just follow. Not to simply look around and see what else might be going on, but to stay in a lane and do the same thing. This blinkered approach leads to a dearth of creativity, with people unable to find an individual voice and carve out their unique style.

It's OK to admire a particular look or style, but trying to replicate it doesn't always work and sometimes requires an advanced skill, and for many it brings frustration. It knocks confidence when people already feel vulnerable and exposed, and leads to the statements of negativity I hear all the time: 'makeup isn't for me', 'I don't suit makeup', 'I can't do it'.

My answer to all of this, and more, is this book. I have always encouraged people to play, to experiment, to learn and enjoy the process. I have worked with thousands of people with very different experiences and skill sets to help them develop their own sense of worth when working with makeup. From professional MUAs (makeup artists) to students, makeup lovers and makeup novices, they all have the same journey: one of learning to play. I've witnessed them having fun discovering new things, and seen them inspired to evolve and develop their own artistry. And I have put all of this experience and knowledge into the book you now hold.

You will not find rules about how you should do something: as it's been said many times before me, there are no rules when it comes to makeup. However, there are some fundamental guidelines which will help you to figure out your own best methods. Think of this book as the 'anti-how to' makeup bible. You will discover how to think beyond the conventional to achieve a look; how to perfect, or sometimes imperfect, classic techniques; how to disrupt the norm. There are no trends to follow here, but what you might find is the inspiration to start a new trend that you've created yourself.

Glowography is not about unachievable beauty standards. It is about finding your own path to a unique and personal identity that can be enhanced and presented to the world via makeup. There are no lists of expensive products you need to buy, and no expensive tools (in fact, we even suggest giving application with a spoon a go). Products are discussed according to how they might potentially be used, according to their texture or colour. Just as in life, it's not about labels – it's about what's inside and how you use it that counts.

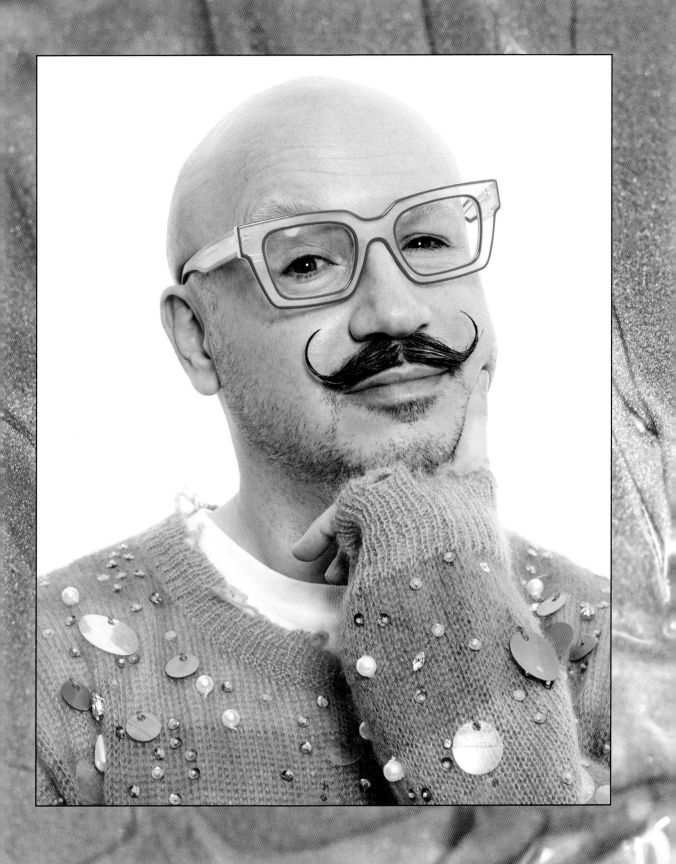

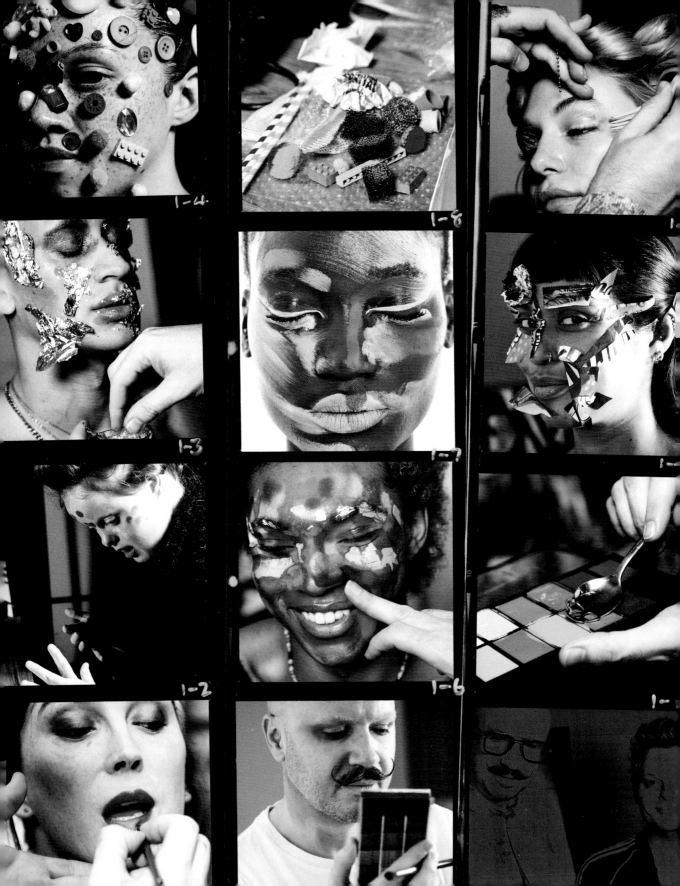

Organised Chaos!

To help you rethink about makeup and creativity, this book is divided into three chapters, 'Experiment', 'Create the Look' and 'Sharpen Your Skills,' all to help with the reprogramming of how you approach makeup. The first chapter encourages you to dive straight in with some unbridled play: create, imagine and make a mess. After you've played, examine the chaos and find the hidden gems within the very happy accidents.

'Create the Look' will help you to expand upon these in order to put together finished looks. Perhaps you'll develop a colour combination you never expected, or notice a chance placement that just seems to work, or maybe you'll have discovered a use for something that never occurred to you before. You might create a big look, a party look, a simple look, or all of the above. It could be something you'd never go out in, or the inspiration for your next big event.

Once you've played and then curated, the final section gives you the opportunity to tighten your new skills. Where most books work on the principle of starting with the basics and building up, I find that never really works due to the confinement and control it creates, instantly squashing any creative potential. I wanted my book to fling the doors of creativity wide open first, allowing you to just play and exercise the creative muscles that we barely get a chance to use. Once these muscles are strong, you can start training them to control the force of the creative explosion and hone your application to achieve your vision. While there are some tips and tricks, these are not intended to tell you what you must do, but provide advice on how you can strengthen what you are doing: how to achieve symmetry if you want it; how to manipulate one product to become something else entirely; how to achieve a smoother blend, etc. Mastering these fundamentals will assist you in elevating your application in your own way.

My hope is that this book allows more people to find their way into makeup, letting them see that it's not just about replication, but that it can be about innovation, and, most importantly, that it's not complicated. Makeup doesn't have to be prescriptive; it can be a tool for self-expression.

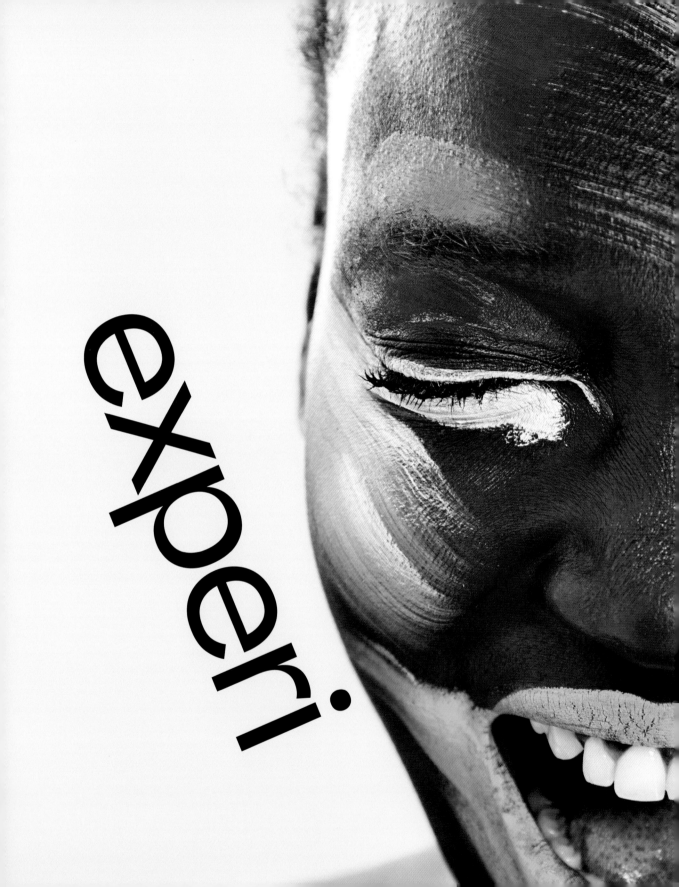

experi

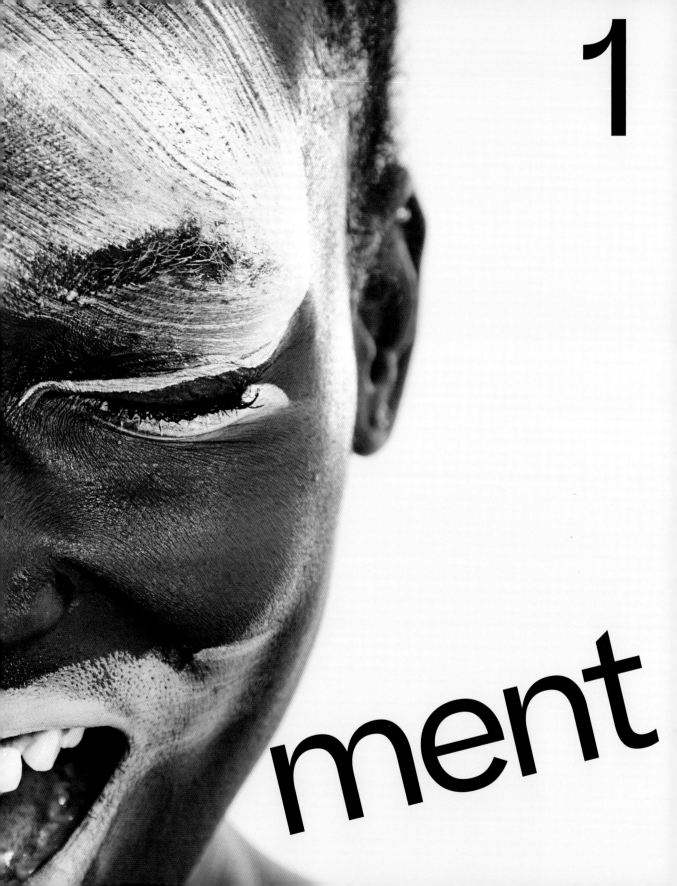

1

ment

I'm often asked where I find inspiration, and the answer is, well, everywhere! Inspiration is all around us. The real question people should be asking is, how do you learn to recognise inspiration? Anyone can discover how to do this, with just a few pointers on which direction to look. This first chapter presents a road map to creative thinking. Creativity is something that, a lot of the time, is stripped from us, because we are first instructed in how to do something 'correctly'. Unfortunately this only serves to build walls that contain and restrict us. We are given the rules of the playground before we are given the ball to play with.

Makeup doesn't need rules, it needs adventure. If you're stuck in a rut and have been doing the same look for years on end, here you will find the crowbar to help you break free. Or perhaps you're a seasoned professional and need some alternative thoughts away from the everyday in order to help bring back the passion or spontaneity. These experiments are here so you can have fun. The purpose is not to end with a finished look: indeed if you do find yourself with a look you'd happily pop to the shops in, then you've done it wrong. This is pure play. Try things out; do something new; force yourself to not care about perfection or worry about the result.

Each experiment presents a challenge to try something new and cast off the restraints that subconsciously hold you back. A lot of the time the experiments will help you to see products in different ways, enabling you to uncover an alternative usage. Makeup products are, at their core, a colour, texture and finish wrapped in a container to aid application, but where it is applied is completely up to you (although you should be mindful of the brand's suggested usage, as items aren't always tested for every eventuality).

You can revisit the challenges again and again, and each time you will come away with a totally different result, learning new things as you go. In true creative spirit, I have carried out these experiments myself with a totally open mind. I have used them in various forms over the years, but rarely have I done them myself. I didn't meticulously plan them out, I had no idea what I was going to end up with, nor what was going to happen along the way. The results are varied, lurching from the totally bonkers to the more problem-solving, with each experiment playing out just as it is shown. They were so much fun to do, and what I loved most was the energy of everyone throughout the process. So get going, and remember to embrace the chaos and enjoy discovering new ways to use makeup.

It's time to raise
the temperature
of colour.

hot

+

cold

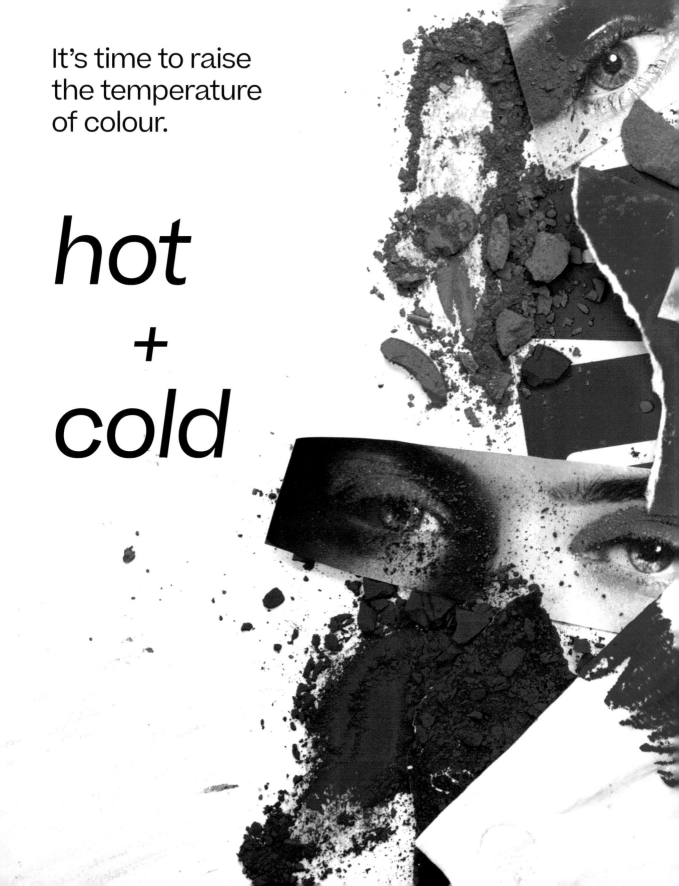

The world is full of colour!

The world is full of colour relationships, and figuring out how different hues work together allows us to make clever choices to get the results we want. The colour wheel enables us to view the full colour spectrum and see how they transition seamlessly from one to another, from yellow to red to blue and back to yellow. One way in which we categorise colours is by temperature: hot and cold. Anything on the red side of the colour wheel is in the 'hot' group, and anything on the blue side is part of the 'cold' group. Yellow sits between the pair: if you add a little red it becomes warm, add a little blue and it becomes cooler.

Here's how you can work out which colour temperature best suits us. For this experiment, paint one of your eyes or your model's eyes blue or another cool colour, and the other red or a different hot colour. Be bold with your application, and wrap the eye in colour, going up towards and over the brow and deep under the eye, touching the orbital bone. Once you've done this, view yourself in the mirror; looking directly into the iris, cover up first one eye and then the other, and you'll be able to see how your own eye colour reacts to the colour that is surrounding it. Does your eye colour calm down or become darker, or does it become intensified and pop, or perhaps even appear to change colour?

DOM SAYS

YOU DON'T HAVE TO USE THE SAME TYPES OR TEXTURES OF PRODUCT: THIS IS ABOUT COLOUR, SO IT DOESN'T MATTER IF ONE IS A CREAM STICK AND THE OTHER IS A POWDER.

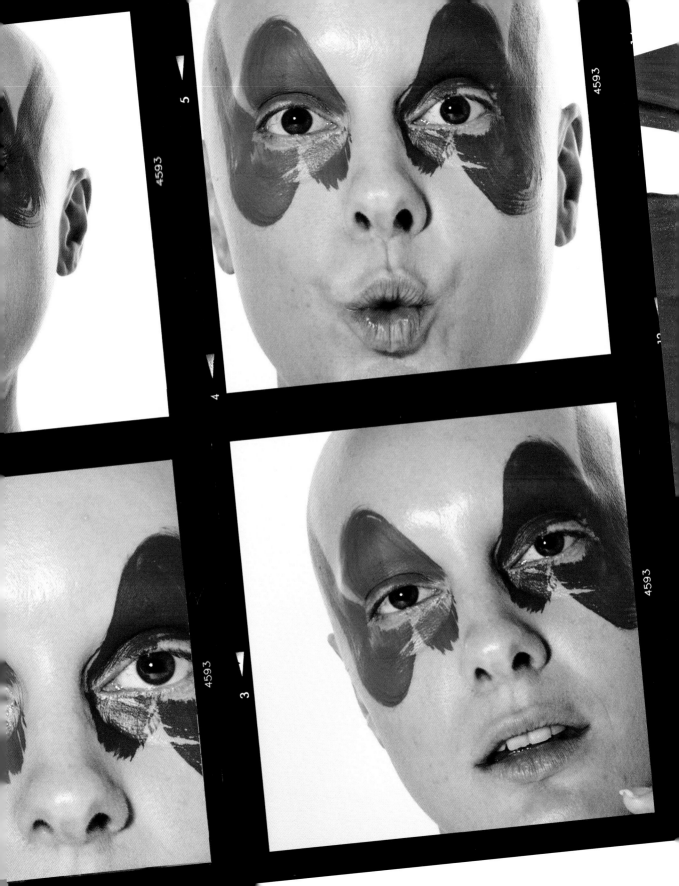

Mono chro me

The pigment power of a single colour.

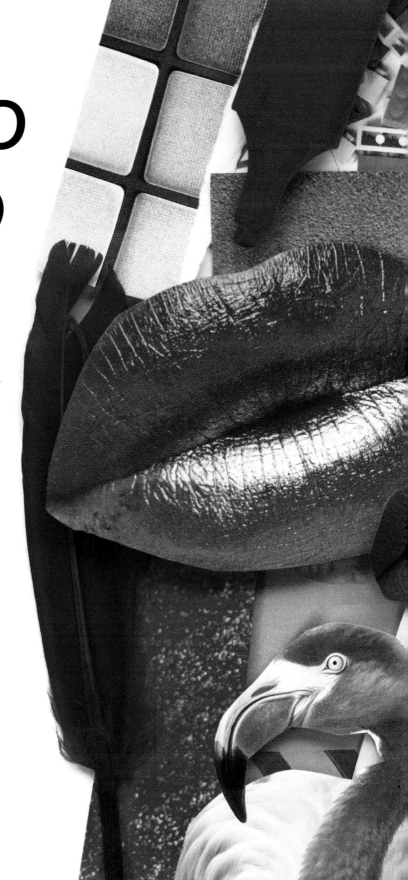

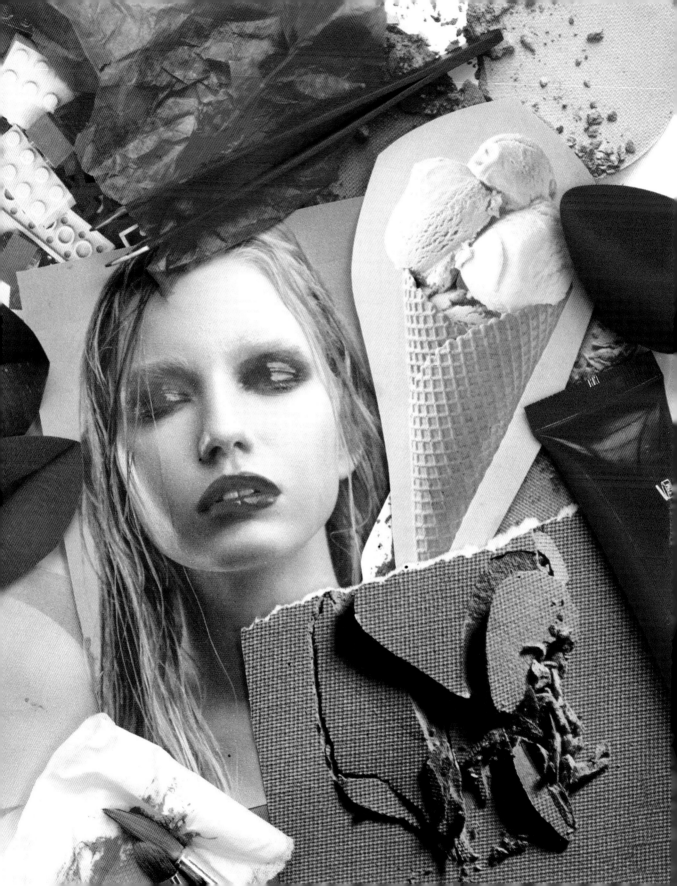

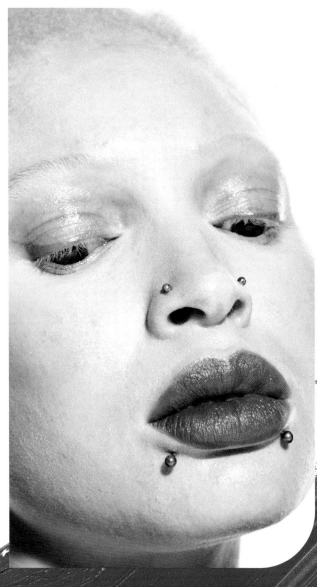

We've touched on colour already, with the simple organisation of colours into hot or cold (p.18), but there's so much more to discover about the technicolour world. Each colour has its own tonal spectrum, varying from light or pale to deep and dark, known as the hue. Any makeup product can deliver different hues simply by varying the amount of pressure you use and how many layers you apply. For a light or pale hue, simply apply the product lightly, or press down to build greater depth of colour.

For this experiment, select one colourful product and use only that in all areas to create a classic makeup look. Alter the pressure of the application to introduce different levels of depth for a balanced look. If, for instance, you use a light wash of colour across the eyes, you may wish to use a more intense amount to create an eyeline. You might apply sheer colour to the cheeks, but then intensify the hue under the cheek bone to give dimension in the form of a contour. You could even think about how you might use it on the brow. Not everything is going to work; this is about discovering how much you can do with a single product.

Not everything is going to work. Discover how much you can do with one product!

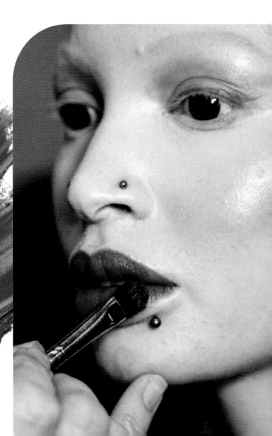

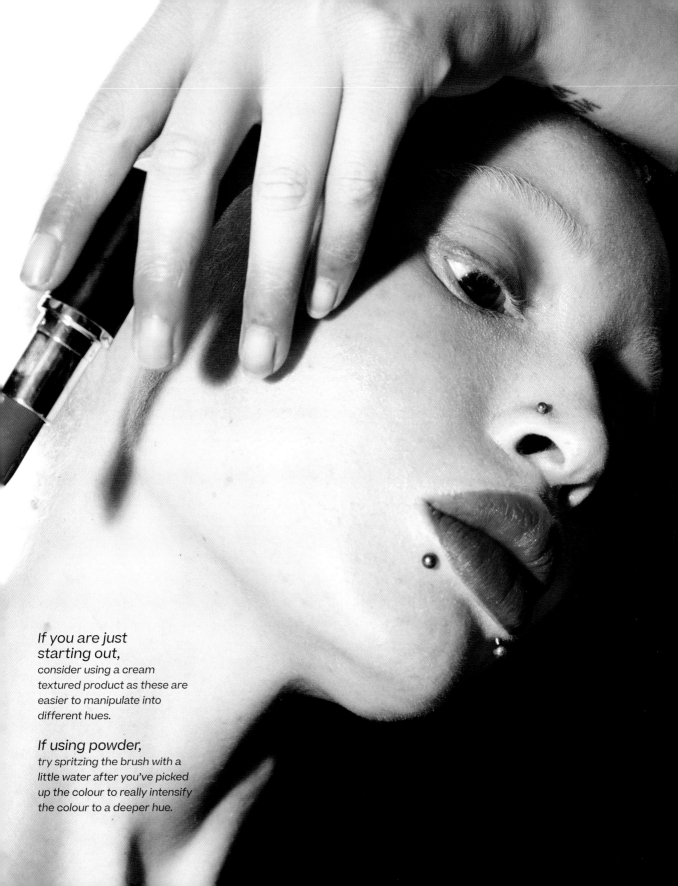

If you are just starting out, consider using a cream textured product as these are easier to manipulate into different hues.

If using powder, try spritzing the brush with a little water after you've picked up the colour to really intensify the colour to a deeper hue.

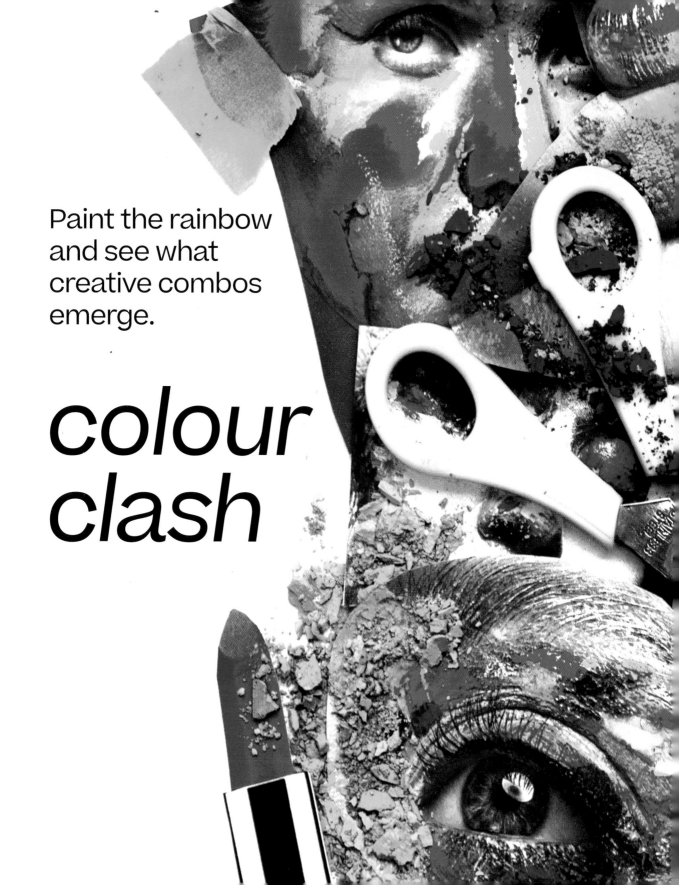

Paint the rainbow and see what creative combos emerge.

colour clash

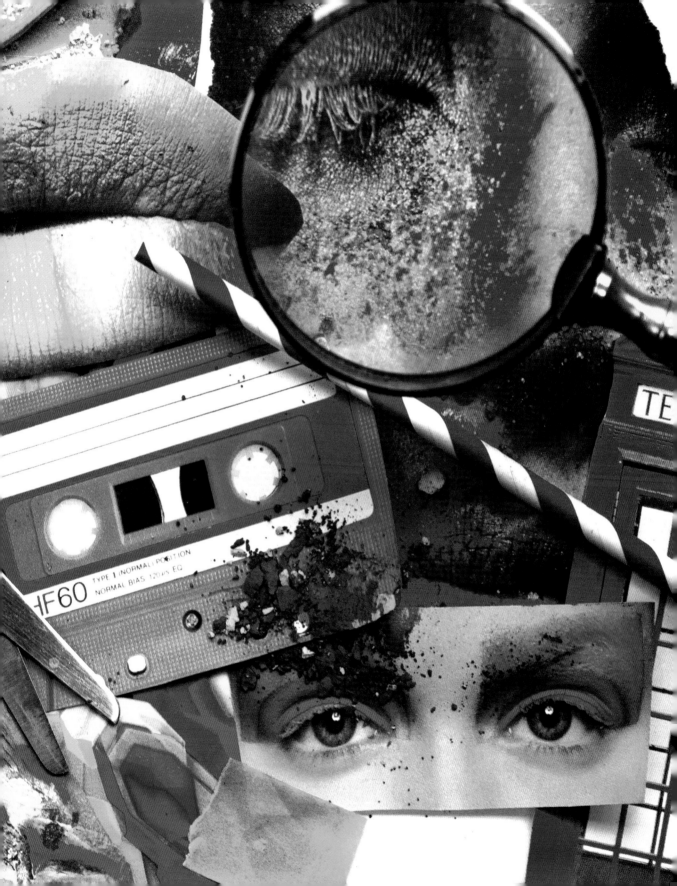

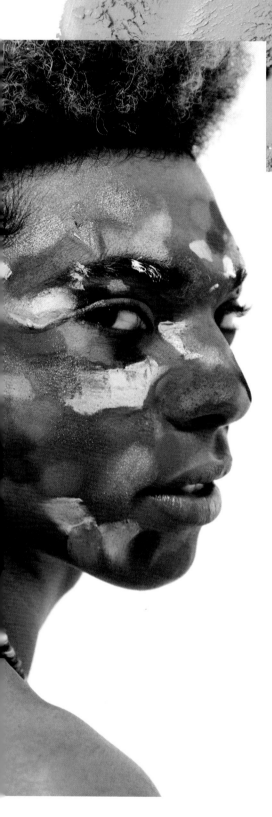

I'm throwing all the doors open to fun!

In the Hot + Cold challenge (p.16), we looked at the temperature of colours, dividing them into hot and cold depending on whether they had a blueish (cool) or reddish (warm) tone, with yellow being somewhere in the middle. Now we'll take it a step further with a quick guide to basic colour theory. The three primary colours (red, blue and yellow) on the colour wheel will enable you to make all other colours; when you mix two primaries together you get secondary colours (green, orange and purple), and these sit between the primaries. Those that sit opposite each other on the wheel (such as purple and yellow, red and green, and blue and orange) are known as complementary colours, and using them together makes each of them really pop.

For this challenge, begin applying one colour, maybe starting around the eye. Now sweep another colour next to it. Once you've filled your lid with colour, keep switching to different colours and go over the brow, down onto the cheekbone, across the forehead, and so on. Don't worry about precise application, this is about instinctively choosing and using colour, so smudge and smear away. Keep going until your whole face is a riot of colours. You can repeat colours from the same palette, making sure that they always lay next to colours that they've never touched before, or move on to a completely different palette or other colourful products.

DOM SAYS

ONCE YOU'VE FILLED THE FACE WITH COLOUR, ZOOM IN AND LOOK AROUND FOR ANY INTERESTING COLOUR COMBOS THAT YOU ARE DRAWN TO.

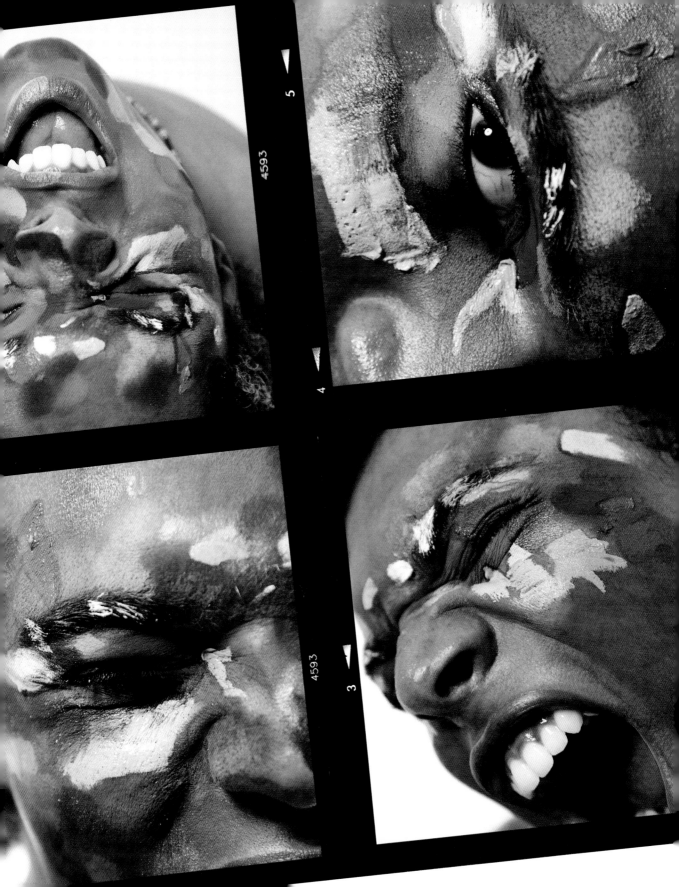

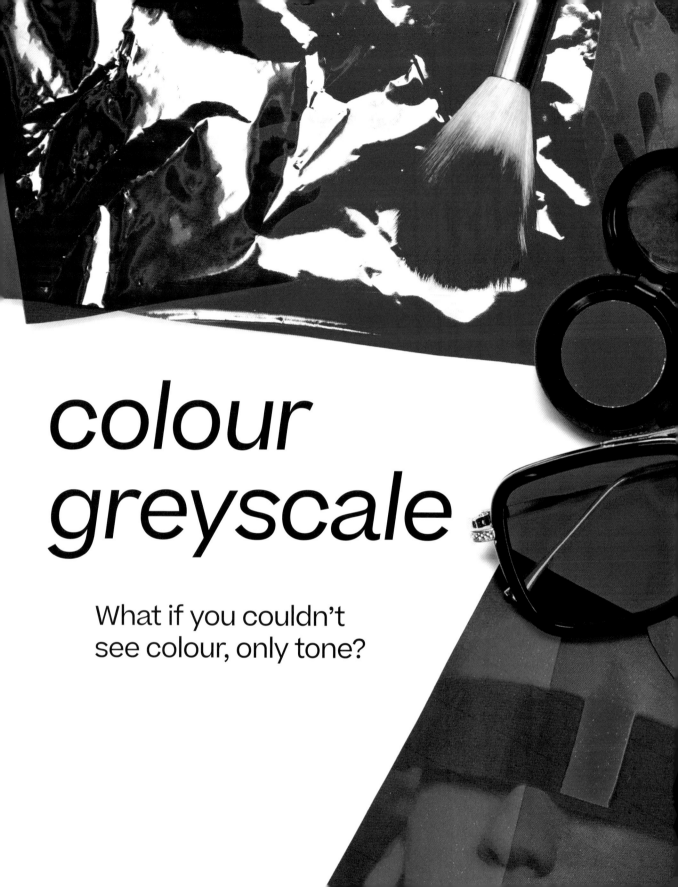

colour greyscale

What if you couldn't see colour, only tone?

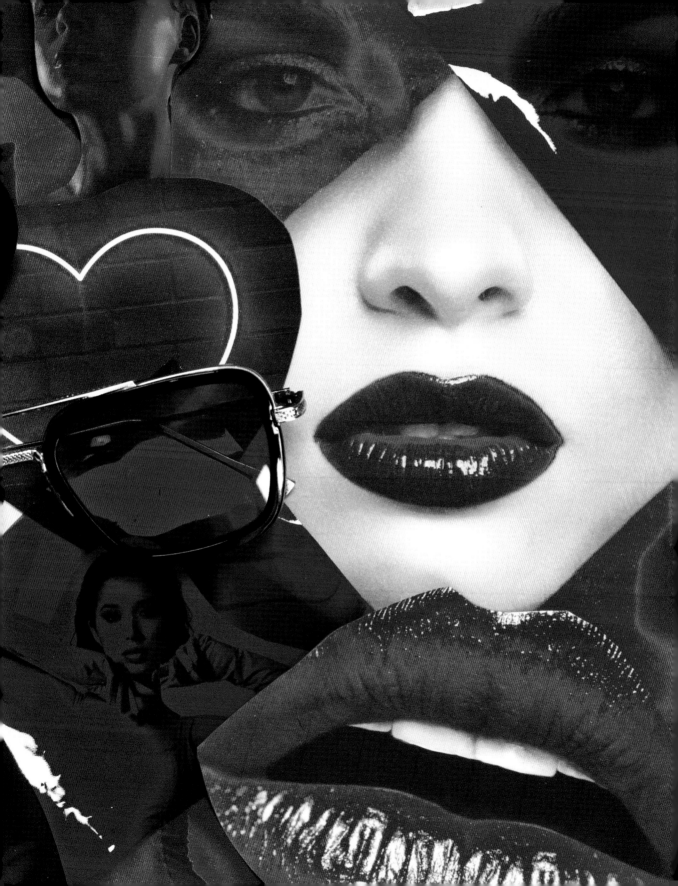

Use the tones and depths of the colours instead.

Colour has always played a huge role in makeup, but did you know it even played a part during the early days of black and white cinema? Makeup artists would paint the faces of actors in different colours to create contrast and definition, helping to emphasise the highlights and contours. They would use bold colours instead of skin tones, because skin tones would be too soft to register and didn't have the sculptural intensity for film. Different colours have different tonal values, meaning some naturally look darker and others lighter. And it was not unusual for lips to be painted green in order to read as red, for example, because the film used at the time caused red to appear black onscreen. If you saw these makeup looks in colour, the crazy results could sometimes be just as stunning.

For this challenge we are going to remove colour from the equation and apply makeup using the tones and depths as our guide. To do this you need to put a coloured gel over a light so that everything in the room turns red, green, blue or yellow. Alternatively, you can use a colour filter on your phone and view the makeup through that as you apply it. Don't read the names on products, and try not to guess what they might be. Once you've completed the look, remove the gel and see what colourful concoction you've created!

DOM SAYS

TRY USING A PALETTE OR PRODUCTS YOU'RE NOT FAMILIAR WITH.

30

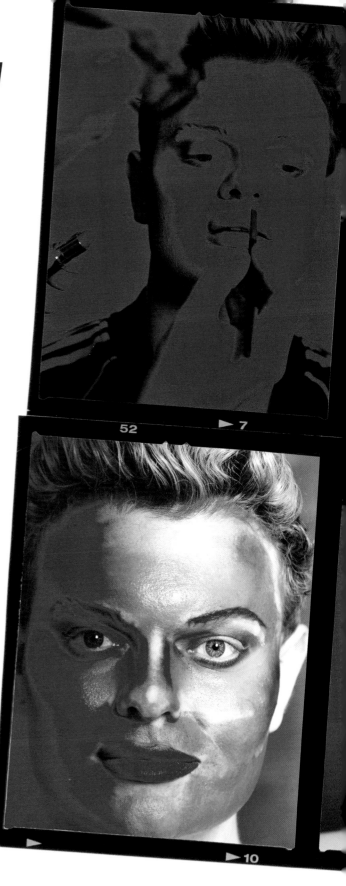

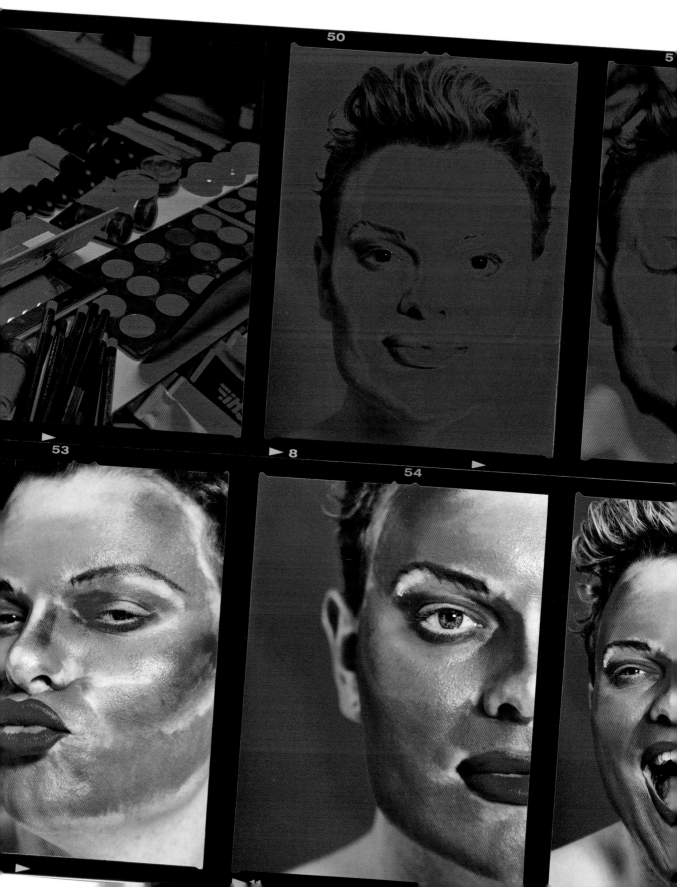

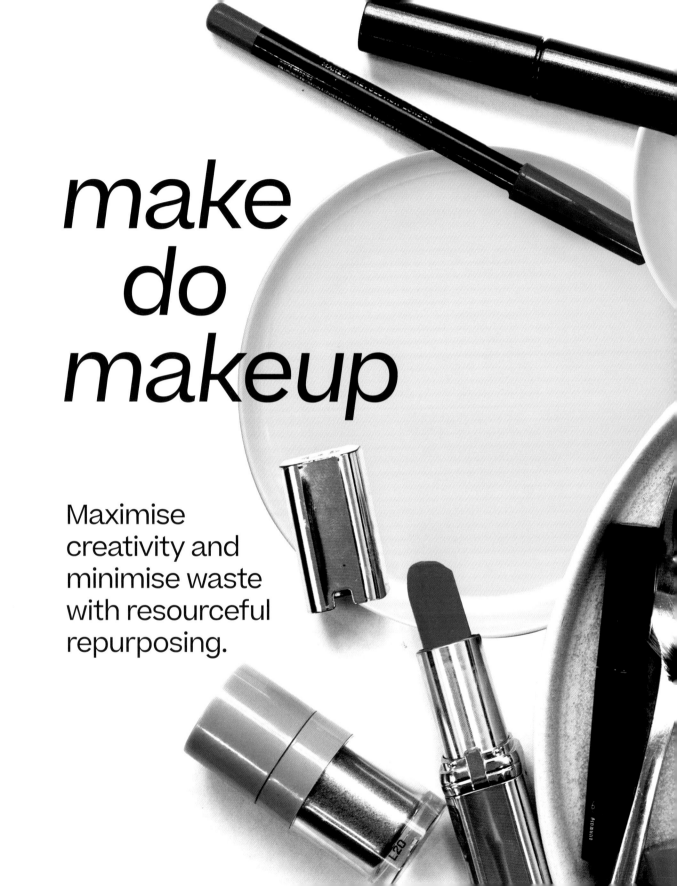

make
do
makeup

Maximise creativity and minimise waste with resourceful repurposing.

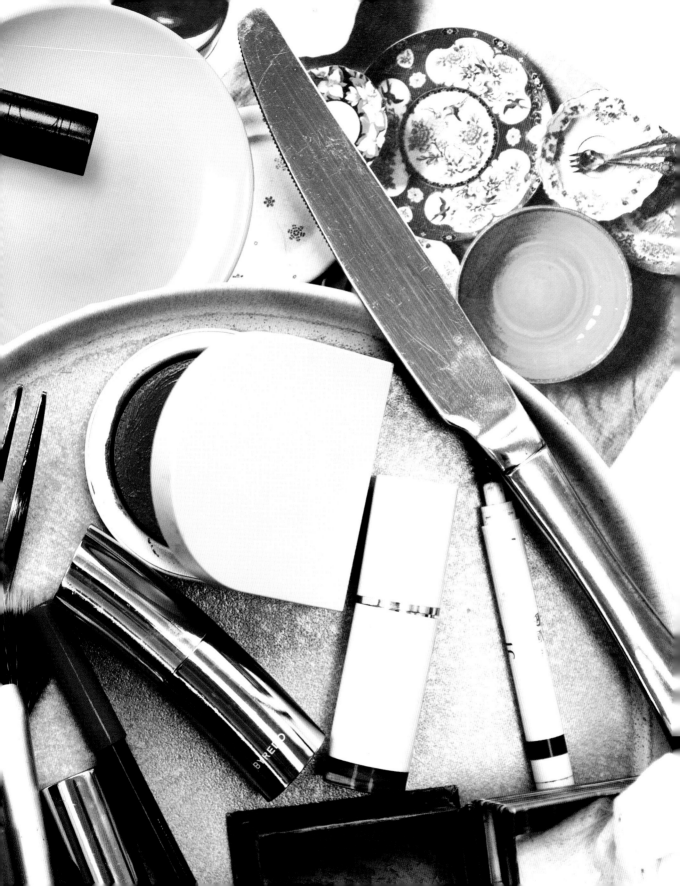

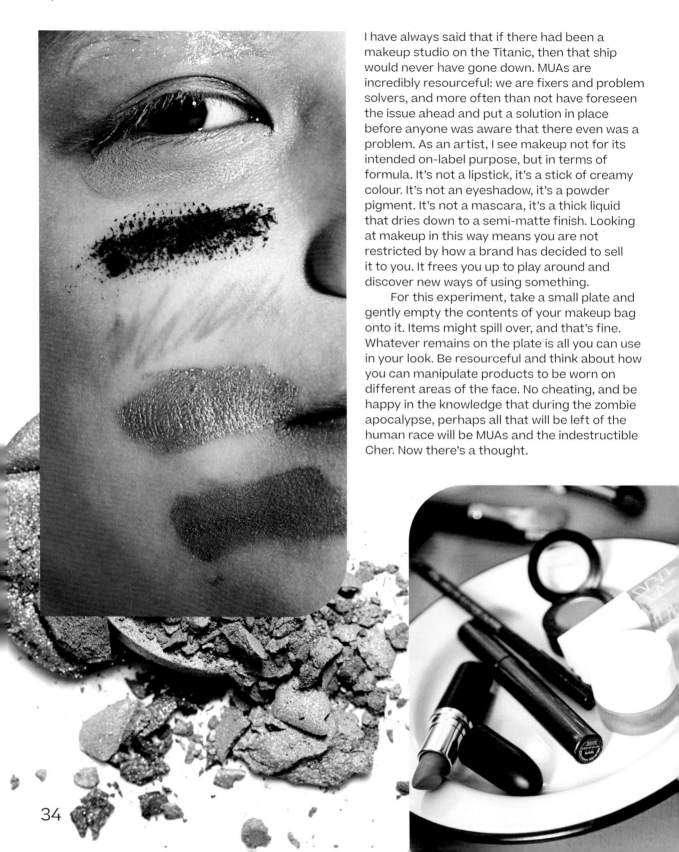

I have always said that if there had been a makeup studio on the Titanic, then that ship would never have gone down. MUAs are incredibly resourceful: we are fixers and problem solvers, and more often than not have foreseen the issue ahead and put a solution in place before anyone was aware that there even was a problem. As an artist, I see makeup not for its intended on-label purpose, but in terms of formula. It's not a lipstick, it's a stick of creamy colour. It's not an eyeshadow, it's a powder pigment. It's not a mascara, it's a thick liquid that dries down to a semi-matte finish. Looking at makeup in this way means you are not restricted by how a brand has decided to sell it to you. It frees you up to play around and discover new ways of using something.

For this experiment, take a small plate and gently empty the contents of your makeup bag onto it. Items might spill over, and that's fine. Whatever remains on the plate is all you can use in your look. Be resourceful and think about how you can manipulate products to be worn on different areas of the face. No cheating, and be happy in the knowledge that during the zombie apocalypse, perhaps all that will be left of the human race will be MUAs and the indestructible Cher. Now there's a thought.

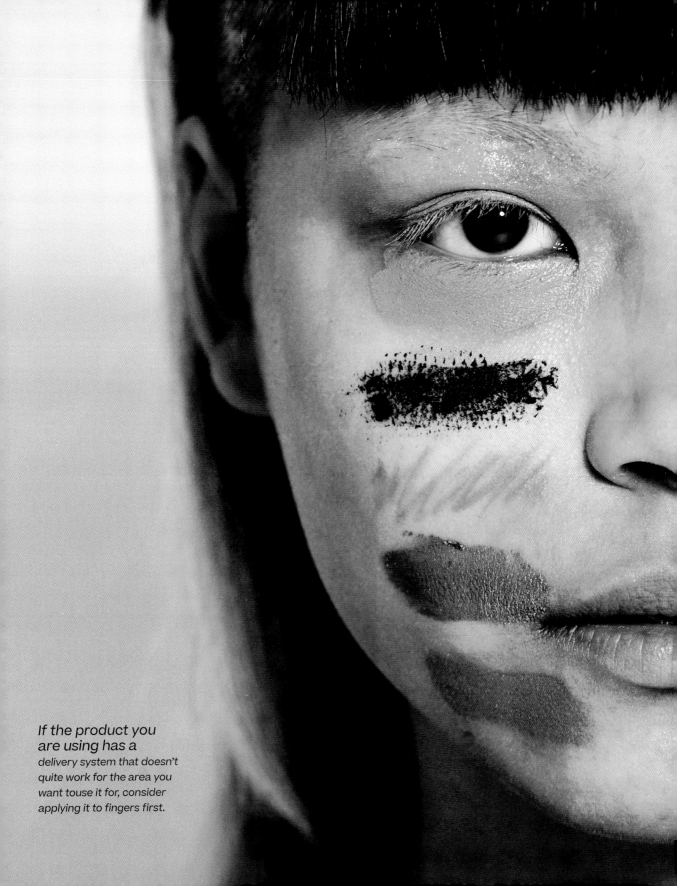

If the product you
are using has a
delivery system that doesn't
quite work for the area you
want touse it for, consider
applying it to fingers first.

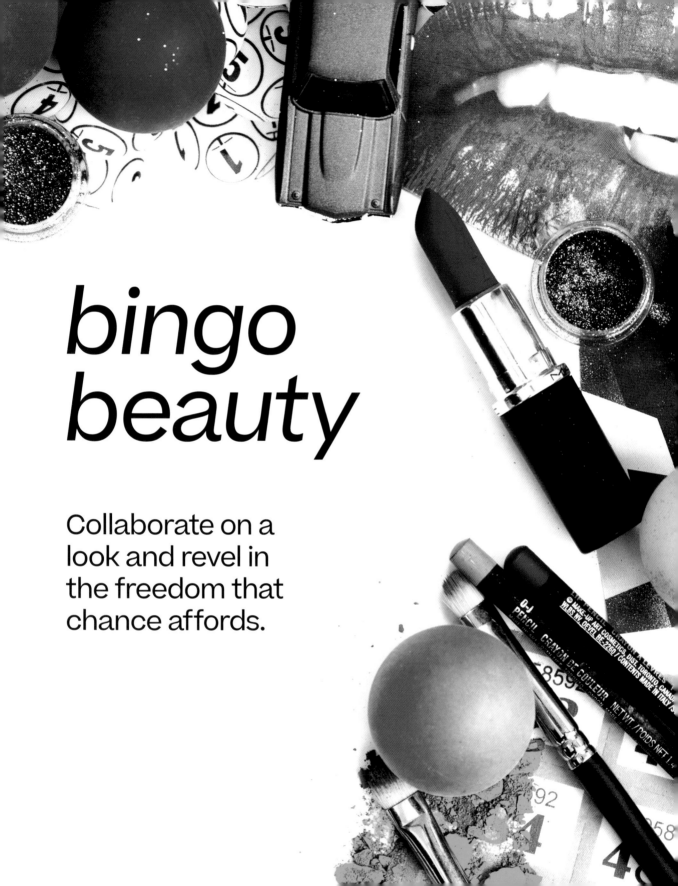

bingo
beauty

Collaborate on a look and revel in the freedom that chance affords.

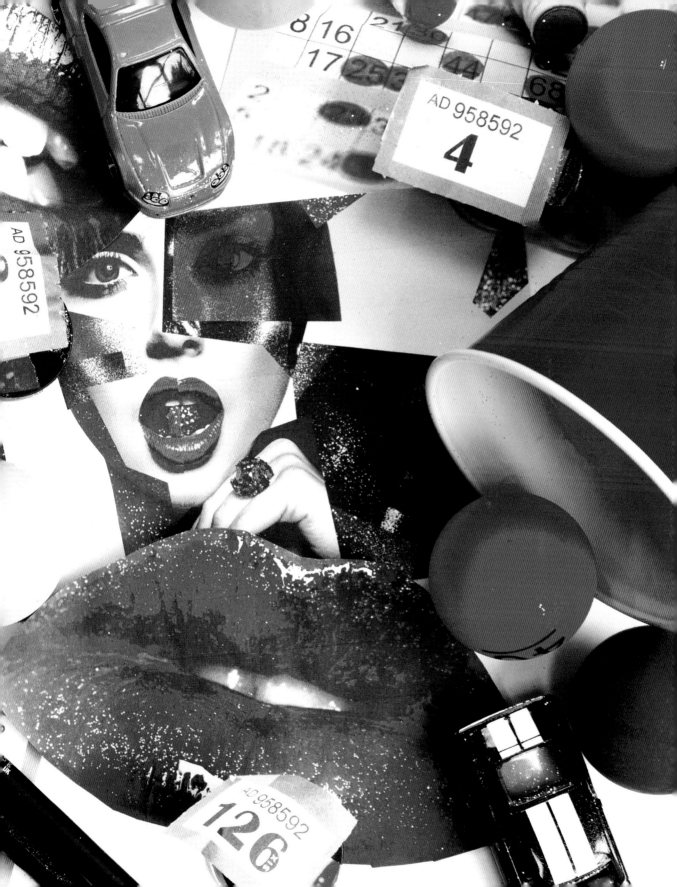

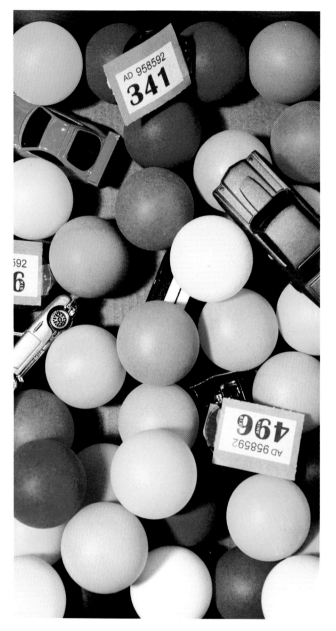

Makeup is a serious business and a respected profession, requiring a diverse set of skills. But let's not forget the most important part: it allows you to be creative and have fun! This challenge is designed to change up your usual makeup routine, test your problem-solving skills, and get rid of the weight of choice so that you can just enjoy makeup!

BINGO BEAUTY

Get out all of your makeup and label it with a number. Maybe skincare is 1–10, foundation 11–20, eyeshadows 21–30, and so on. Now ask someone to give you a number from each of these groups, or ask in a group chat for everyone to give you 1 or 2 numbers from 1 to however many products there are. You will then use these numbered products in your look.

CALL A FRIEND

Ask a friend to pick two or three colours from a makeup palette, selecting an eye pencil, lip colour and either highlighter, blusher or bronzer (or all three). You can also get them to randomly decide where you will use each item. To make this even more of a challenge, find someone who knows nothing about makeup to make the choices, and see how you fix up.

LET FATE DECIDE

Ask the world around you. Put sticky notes on different palettes and label with the names of colours, and whichever colour vehicle passes next decides the one you will use. Open the palette and put those same notes along the rows of colours, and again, whichever car comes along decides on the colour. Or try going by songs on the radio (girl band, boy band, female vocalist, 80s song), or TV ads (food, cleaning, clothing, bank).

Try and do these challenges for a week, see the chaos and randomness unfold.

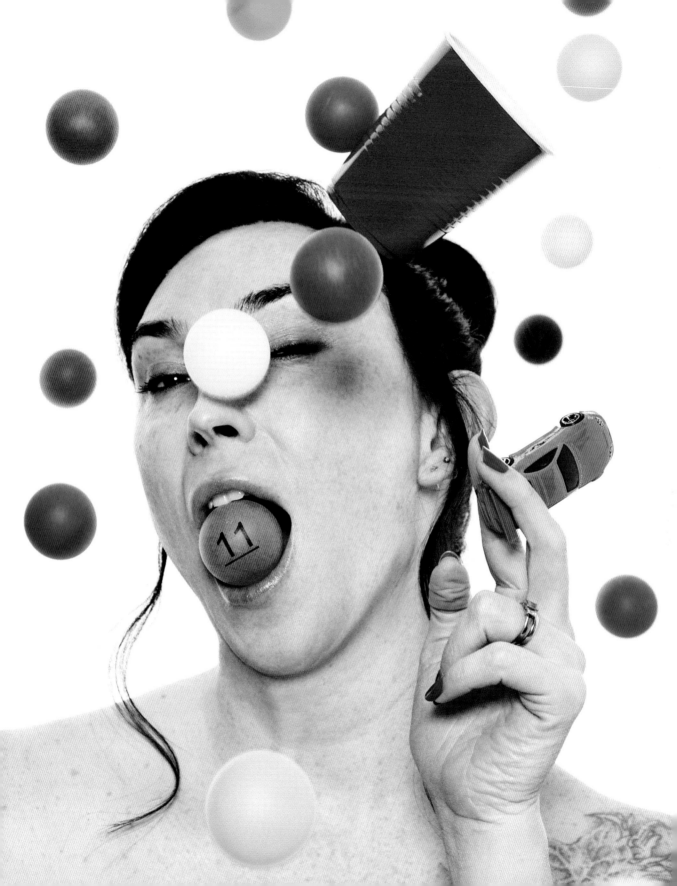

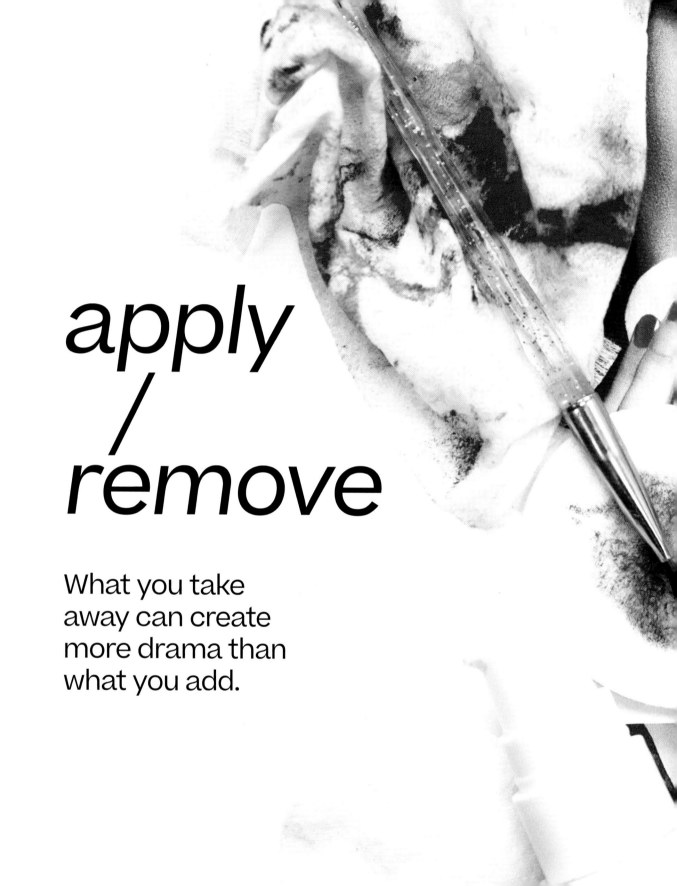

apply
/
remove

What you take
away can create
more drama than
what you add.

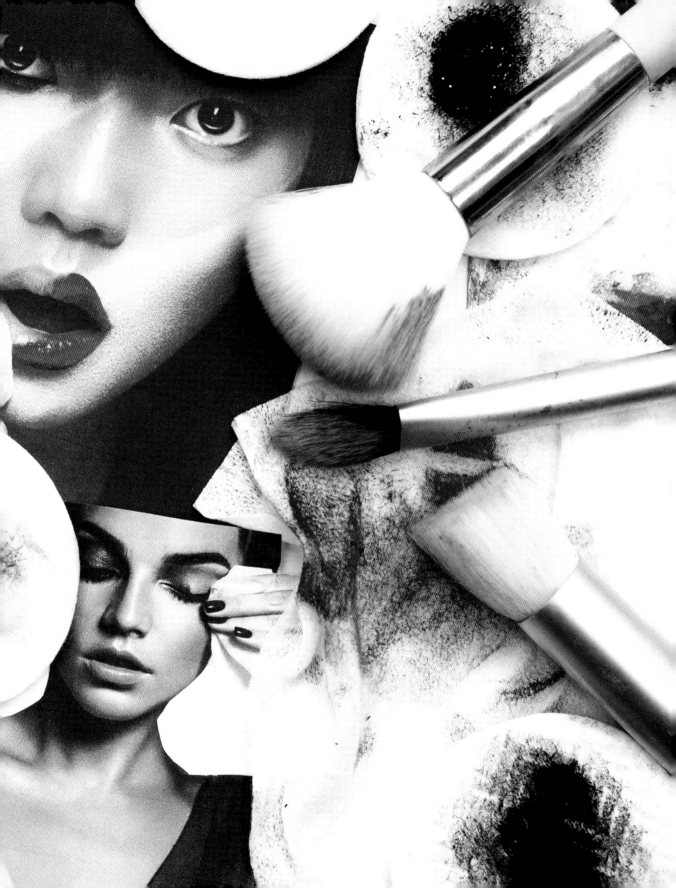

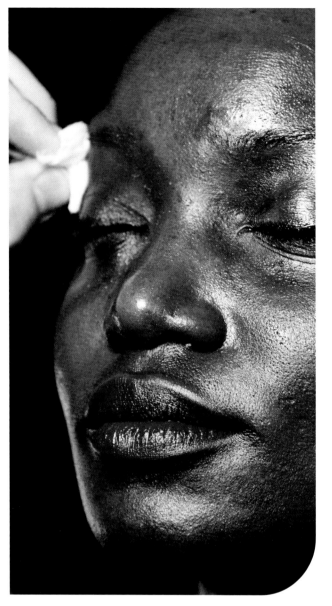

One of the most interesting parts of the makeup process can occur at the end of the day, when you are removing the makeup from yourself or a model. There can be moments when something is only partially cleaned off and maybe mushed together, creating an interesting effect that's exciting to look at, and occasionally the makeup on the wipe is more beautiful that when it was on the face. These effects are the premise for this fun experiment.

Start by applying all the colours in an eyeshadow palette to the eyes. This doesn't have to look good or be symmetrical, and you could put different colours on each eye. Do the same with the cheeks, applying a few different blushers, then move on to the lips. Once you have fully made up the face you can begin removing, but think about different ways of doing this: try scrunching up a cotton pad, pressing down and twisting it into the makeup; use cotton buds dipped in makeup remover to carve out patterns; perhaps apply cleanser to the cheeks and then use a tissue to soak it up and mottle the blushers. Lip colour could be blotted down or partially rubbed off. The idea is to look at how the makeup blends and mixes together while also losing some of the density of pigment.

The idea is to look at how the makeup blends and mixes together while also losing some the density of pigment.

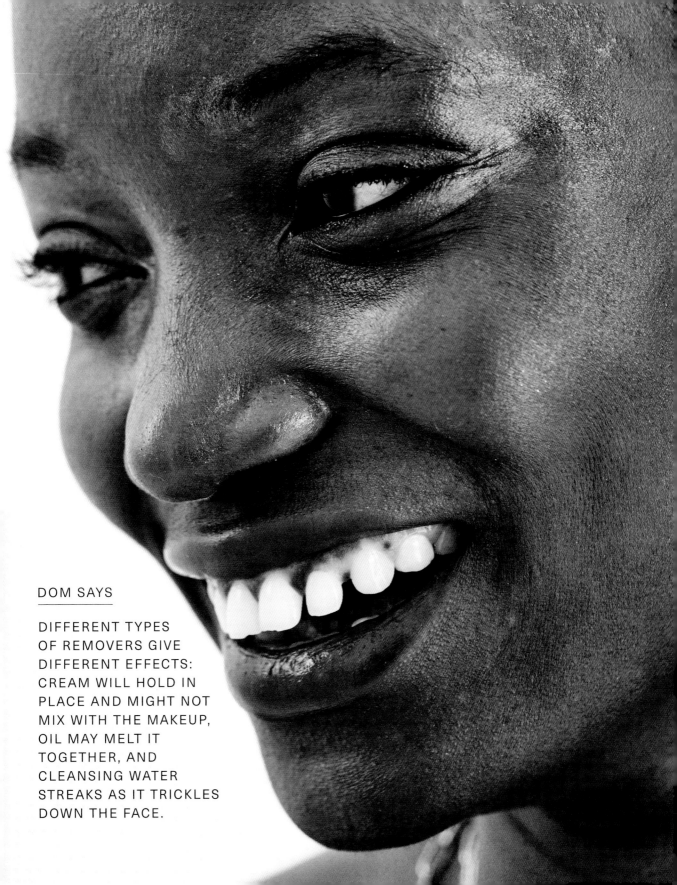

DOM SAYS

DIFFERENT TYPES
OF REMOVERS GIVE
DIFFERENT EFFECTS:
CREAM WILL HOLD IN
PLACE AND MIGHT NOT
MIX WITH THE MAKEUP,
OIL MAY MELT IT
TOGETHER, AND
CLEANSING WATER
STREAKS AS IT TRICKLES
DOWN THE FACE.

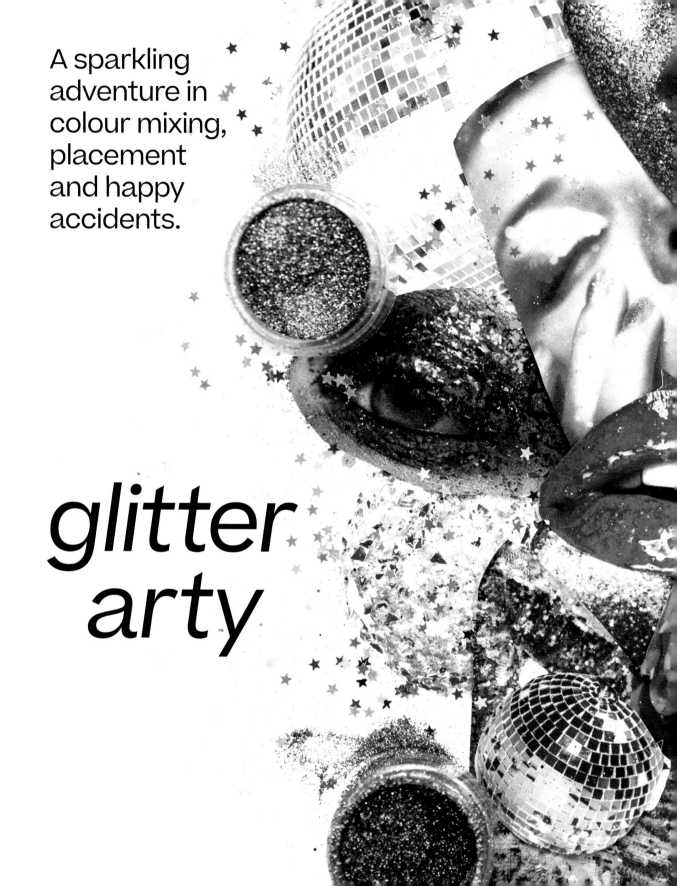

A sparkling adventure in colour mixing, placement and happy accidents.

glitter arty

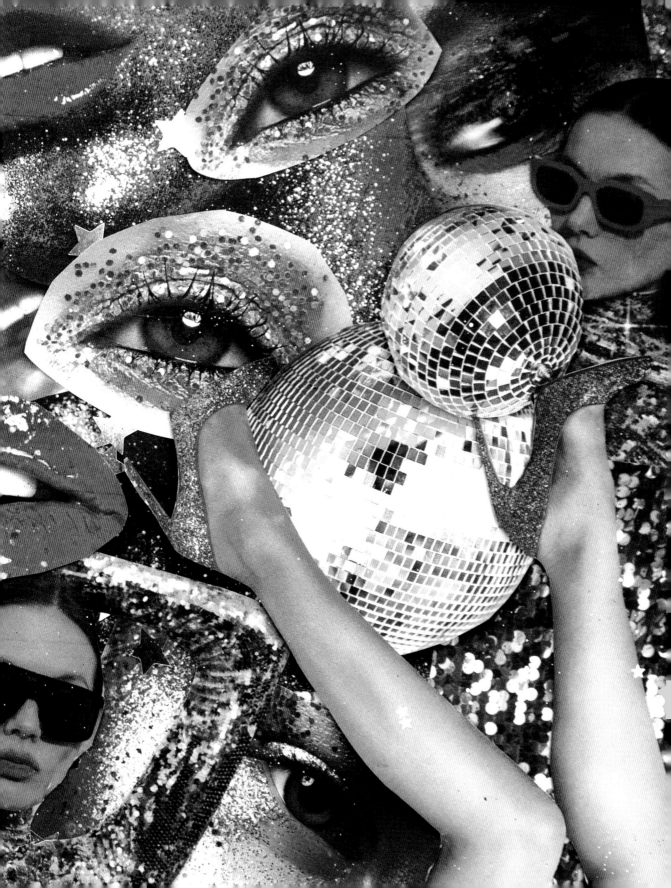

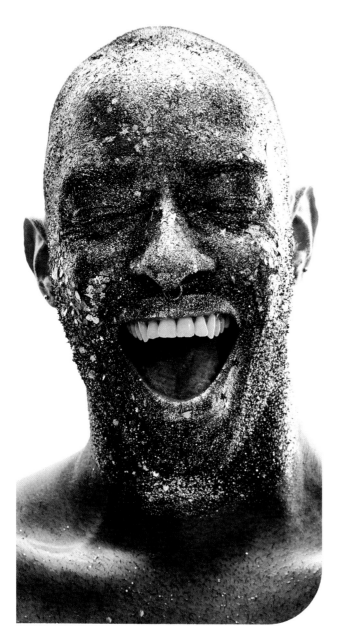

As a fresh-faced makeup artist I remember wanting to dive straight into the glitter and stick it everywhere, but I was never allowed to. Glitter is the ultimate fun product to use in a look, but it felt like I had to focus on a clean base or a 'no makeup' makeup look – all while this shiny pot of magic glinted at the corner of my eye, whispering, 'use me!'

I'm throwing open the doors to the fun cupboard and letting you dive straight in. I want you to grab as many different glitters as you have to hand and sprinkle a little of each onto a plate or a piece of paper. It doesn't matter which colours go where or if they mix or layer, as you'll next use the handle end of a makeup brush to swirl them together. Now get creative applying it to the face: use a cotton bud to add glitter freckles; press it on the lips over clear gloss; draw squiggles all over the face; create glitter tears using a fine brush and lash adhesive, or apply glitter only on the eyebrows for a bold look. Remember to use cosmetic grade glitters if you are going to apply any of the sparkle around the eyelash area. If not, then leave the eye area alone and use powders of cream in similar colours to help with the experiment. Use fingers, sponges, a cotton swab or brush (a dense or flat one will give you more control than a fluffy brush). You could even just close your eyes and roll your face over the paper, letting the glitter stick where it wants to. Don't overthink it!

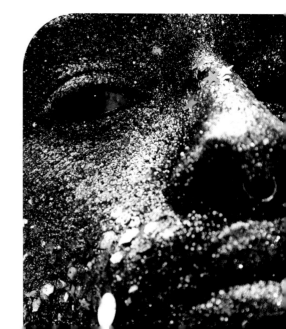

Now, do you dare go grab a pint of milk in this fabulous look?

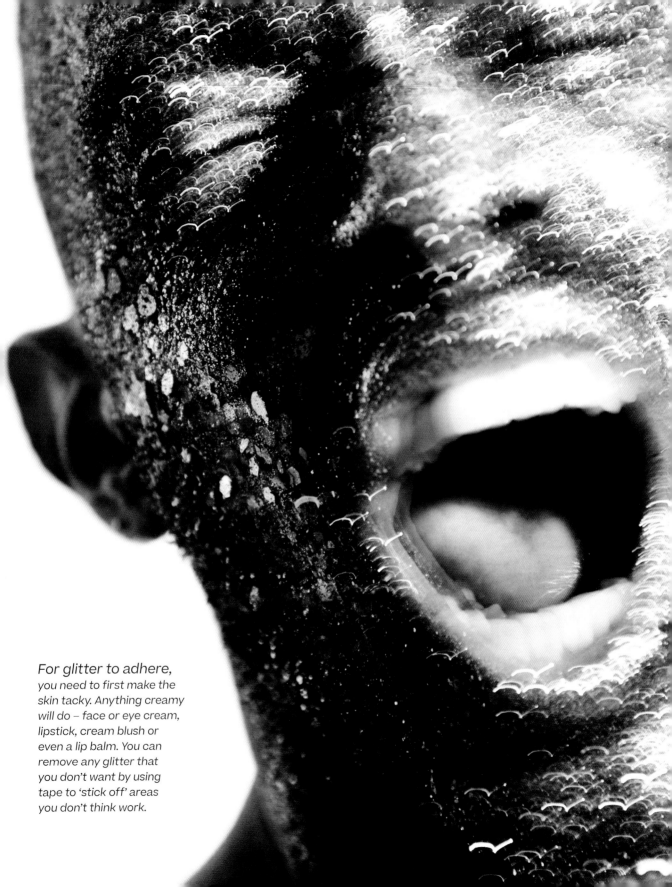

For glitter to adhere, you need to first make the skin tacky. Anything creamy will do – face or eye cream, lipstick, cream blush or even a lip balm. You can remove any glitter that you don't want by using tape to 'stick off' areas you don't think work.

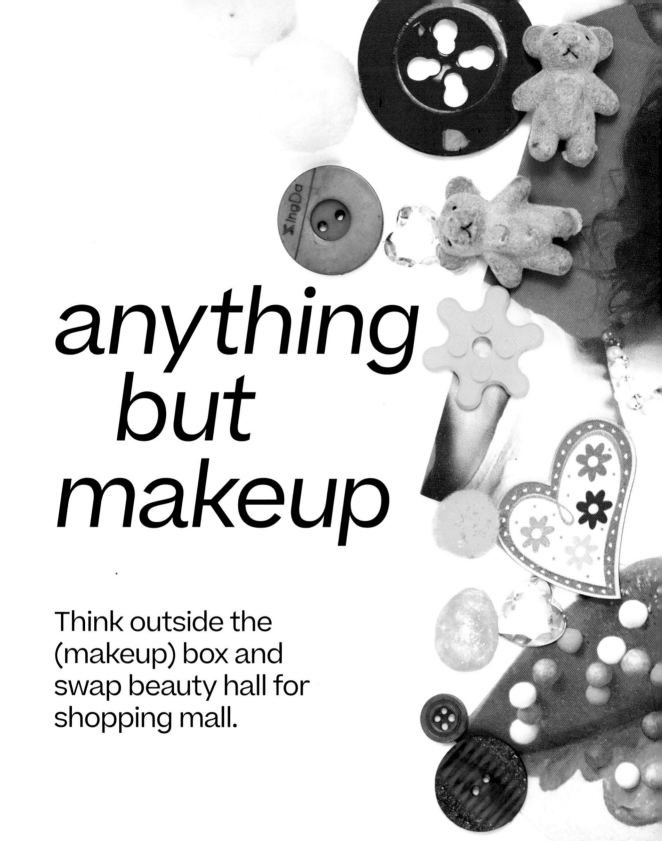

anything but makeup

Think outside the (makeup) box and swap beauty hall for shopping mall.

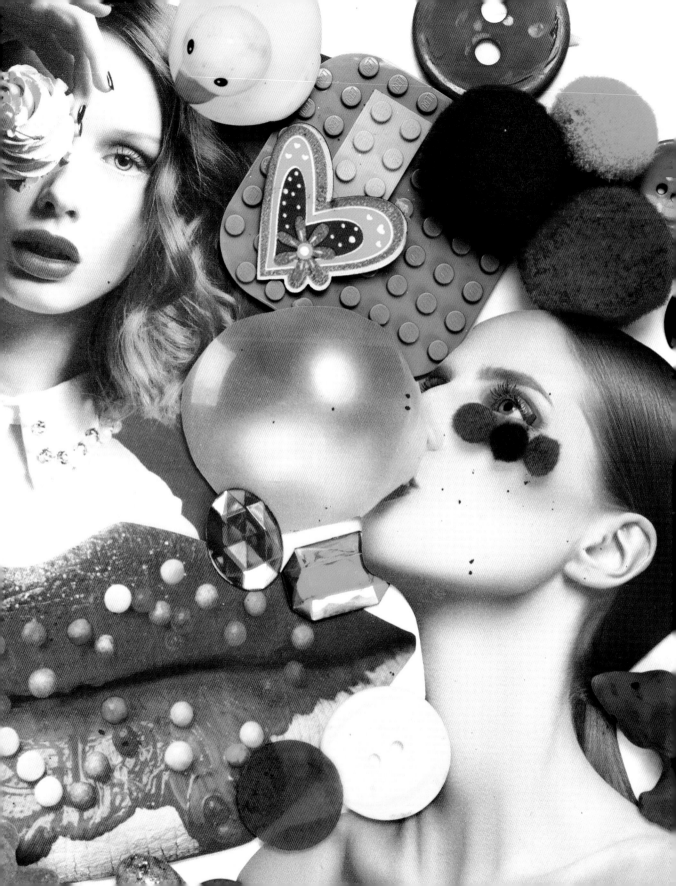

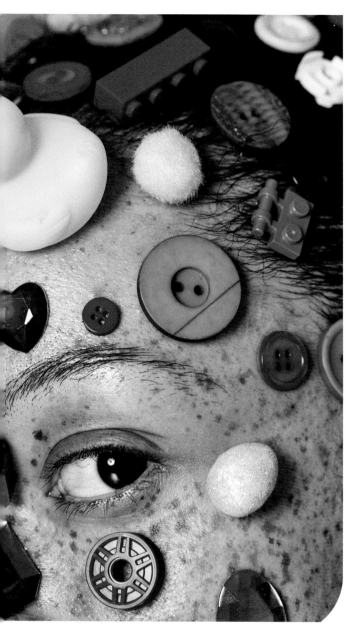

Makeup comes in many different forms, and it doesn't have to be from behind a cosmetics counter. I get excited and inspired about ways to decorate the face whether I'm visiting an art gallery, working a fashion show, or just out shopping. I especially love a stationery store: not just the regular run-of-the-mill office supply chain, but those that sell everything from interesting pens and papers to ribbon and kitsch bits. Throw in some confetti packets and table sprinkles and I'm in heaven.

One of my favourite places in the makeup room is my 'odds 'n' sods' cupboard. It's full of random things I've collected over the years, stuff I decided might one day make for a great look: miniature gravel from a doll's house emporium; a box of random buttons from a thrift store; bags upon bags of confetti. These can be a lot cheaper than buying stickers and templates from a specialist makeup shop, and are a lot more fun and colourful. For this look I would love for you to just raid your odds and sods cupboard or that drawer or shoe box that's filled with knick-knacks and use anything you might have: buttons, beads, even a rubber duck and just cover the face. You could even sprinkle something onto a surface, apply cream or gloss to your face and roll your face into the pile and see what sticks! Consider interesting placements and non-conventional pieces.

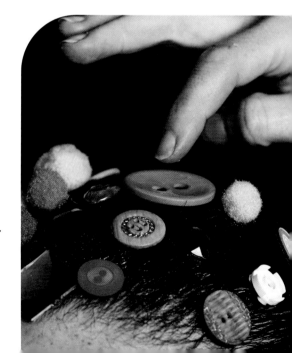

Consider interesting placements and non-conventional pieces.

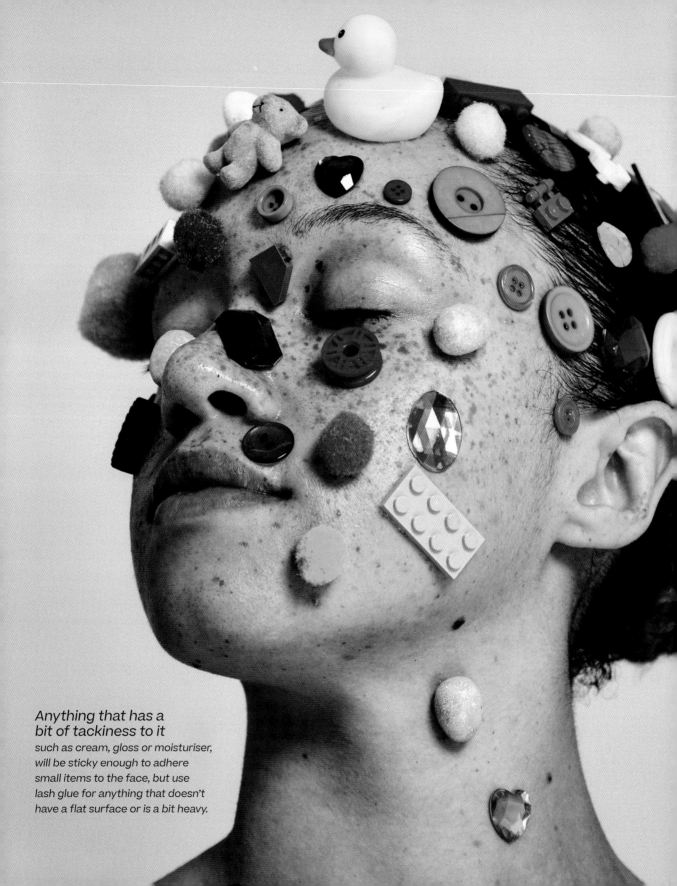

Anything that has a
bit of tackiness to it
*such as cream, gloss or moisturiser,
will be sticky enough to adhere
small items to the face, but use
lash glue for anything that doesn't
have a flat surface or is a bit heavy.*

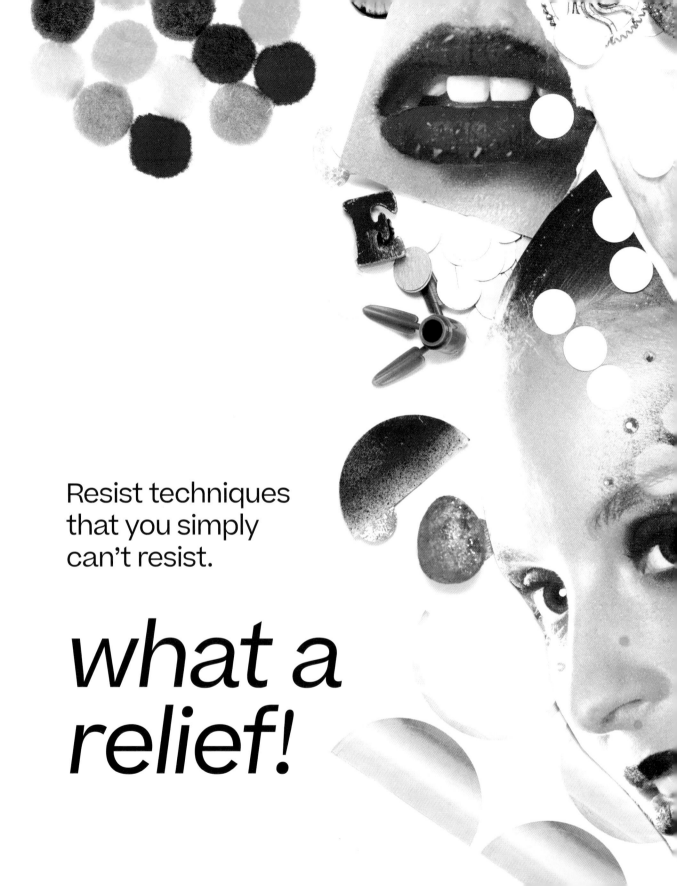

Resist techniques
that you simply
can't resist.

*what a
relief!*

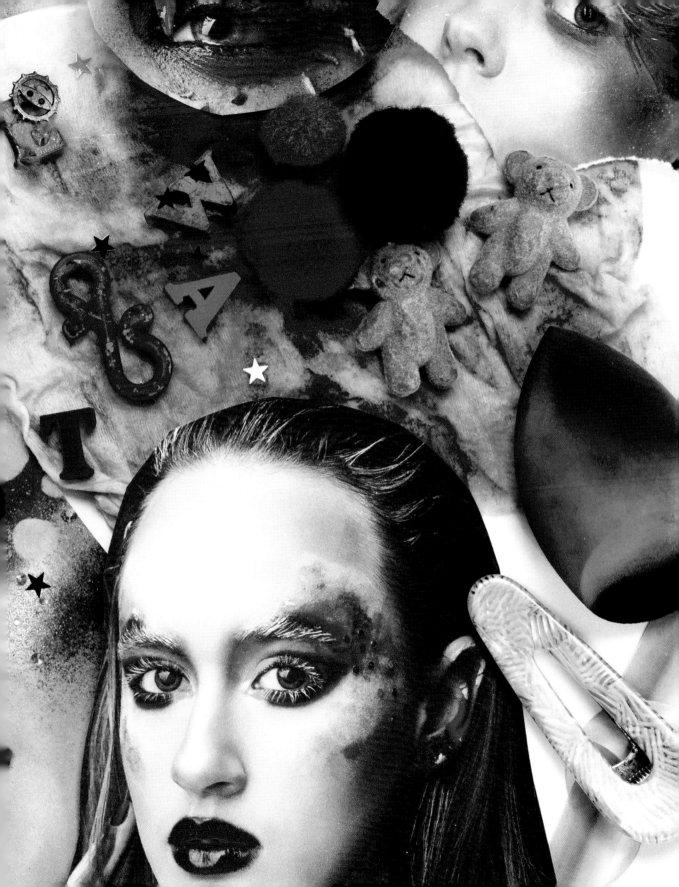

Embellishments like confetti can be used for more than sticking to the face, they can also be great as a sort of stencil. Many years ago, on a work trip, I was performing repeated makeup demonstrations. This started out fun, but after applying the same look over and over, both the model and I were bored, which the audience picked up on. I had been told to stick to the script, but I wanted to be inspiring and give the audience something to get excited about. Looking around during the fifth or sixth class, I noticed a floral display. After I had completed the required look, I took a flower and held it against the model's cheek, then applied eyeshadow to a big fluffy brush and stippled around the edge to reveal the shape of the petals. This simple technique got a great response, so I carried on, using all the colours from the palette to dust around the flower, overlapping them and repeating around the model's face.

This is what we are now going to experiment with, using confetti or any other items you might have used in the Anything But Makeup challenge (p.48). Use a dab of lash glue to apply differently shaped pieces to a clean, moisturised face. Then, using fluffy brushes of varying sizes, apply powder or cream colours all over the face. Once you're done, remove the pieces to expose the skin beneath. You could leave the cut-out shapes bare, apply foundation, or fill them with other colours entirely.

DOM SAYS

WHEN USING LASH GLUE, APPLY A DOT OF GLUE TO BOTH THE CONFETTI AND THE SKIN AND LEAVE TO DRY BEFORE PLACING THEM TOGETHER. LASH GLUE IS A BONDING ADHESIVE SO WILL FASTEN BETTER IF STUCK TO ITSELF WHEN DRY.

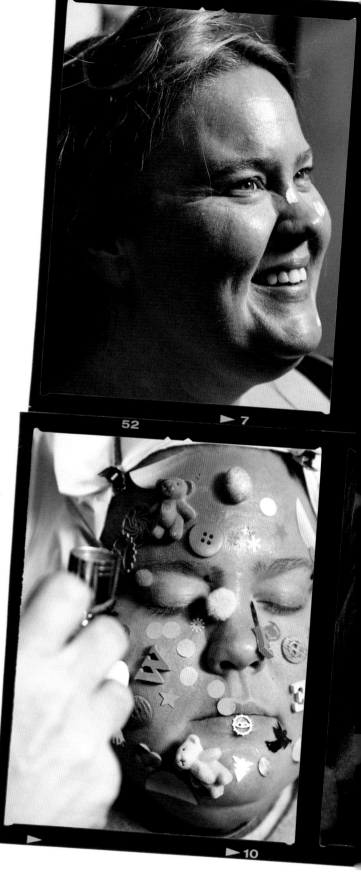

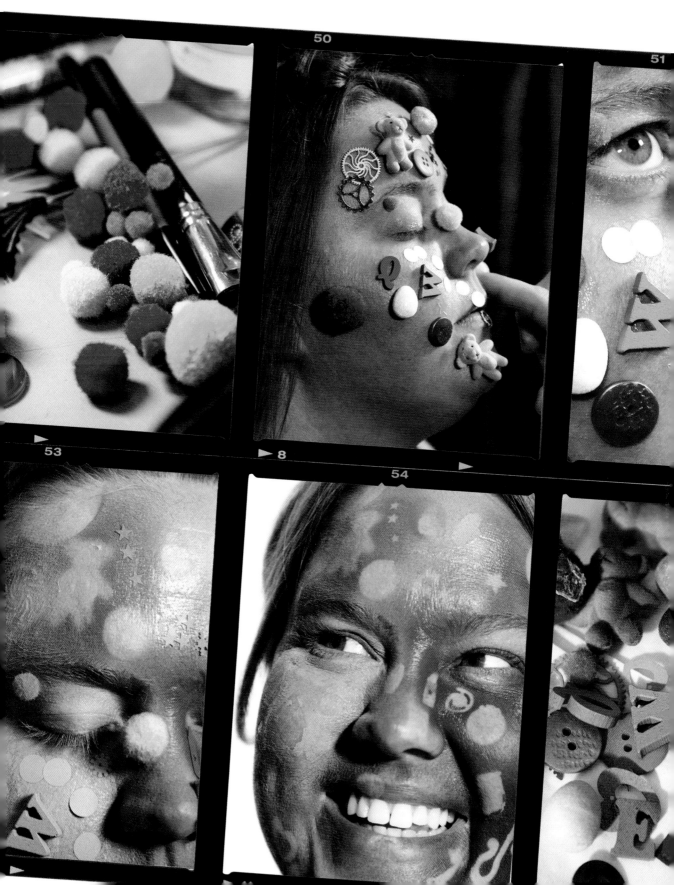

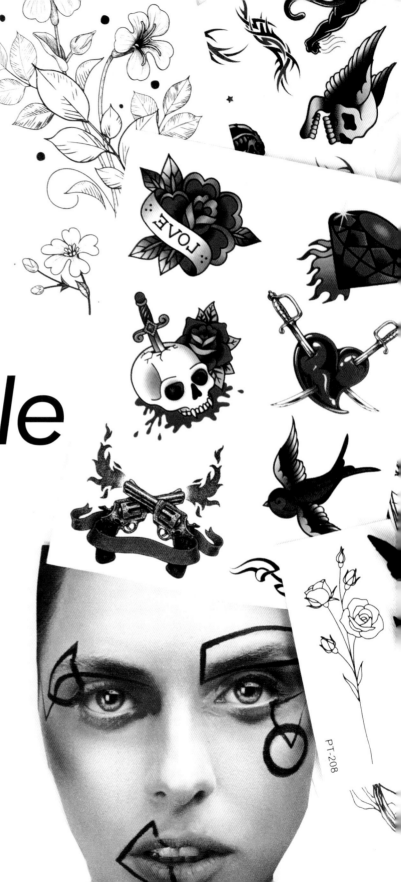

tatt-doodle

Transfer
techniques
for decorative
designs.

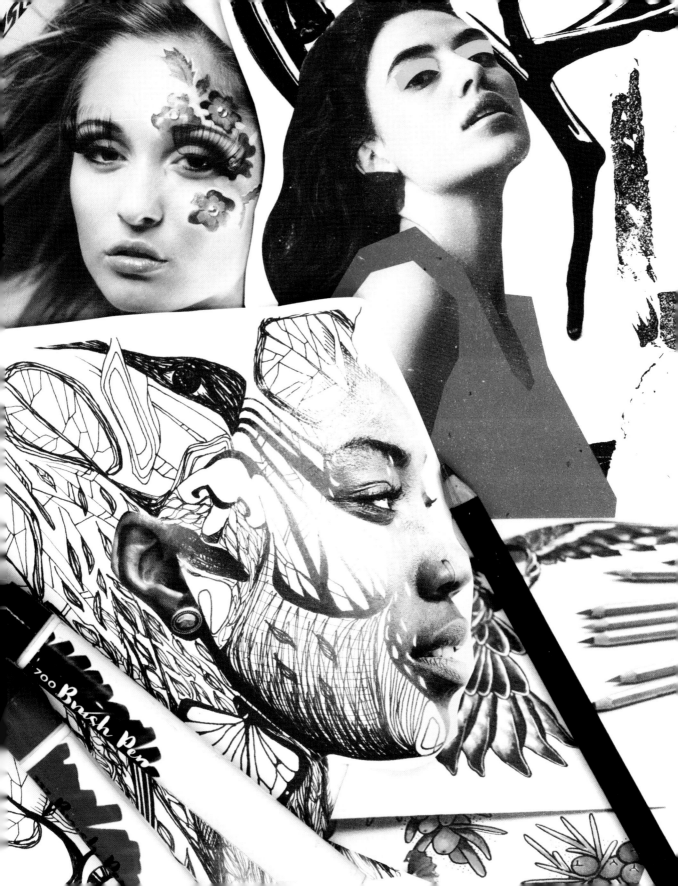

700 Brush Pen

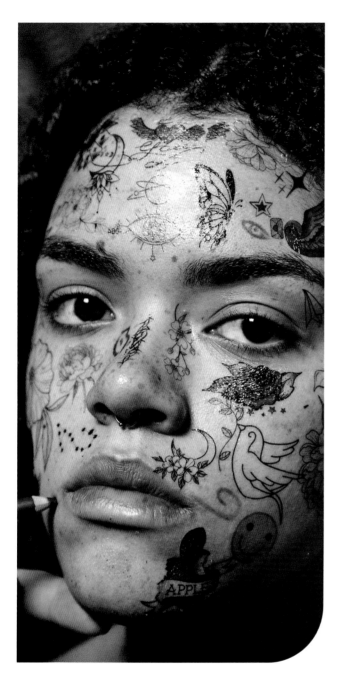

One of my first memories of playing around with makeup was making a paste with my mum's favourite talc and water. I always loved sci-fi, and was obsessed with one of the TV big shows of the 80s called *V*, which featured lizard-like aliens, giant spaceships and laser pistols. I discovered that mixing water with talc made a paste which, when dried, resembled lizard scales. This idea of taking ordinary things from around the house to create magical effects amazed me. Roll on 15 years and I was at university being shown how a Sharpie, baking paper and a deodorant stick could create a tattoo. Today you can purchase 'tattoo paper', which enables to use your home printer to copy out any design you want: it could be an outline of a photo, a doodle from a tablet or a piece of art you've created in a different medium. There are also tattoo pens to draw straight onto the skin. And don't forget more traditional makeup like eye pencils and eye liners. Whatever you use, powder this down to set it, and then add shading, colour or even glitter to decorate. You're not recreating a tattoo as such, this is about transferring big designs onto the face more easily than drawing them freehand.

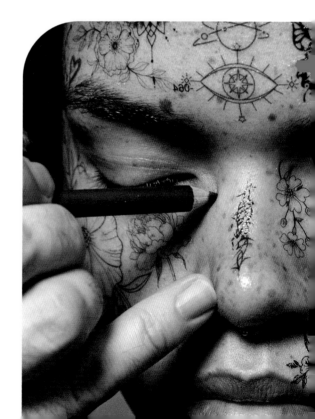

DOM SAYS

THE IDEA OF TAKING ORDINARY THINGS FROM AROUND THE HOUSE TO CREATE MAGICAL EFFECTS AMAZED ME.

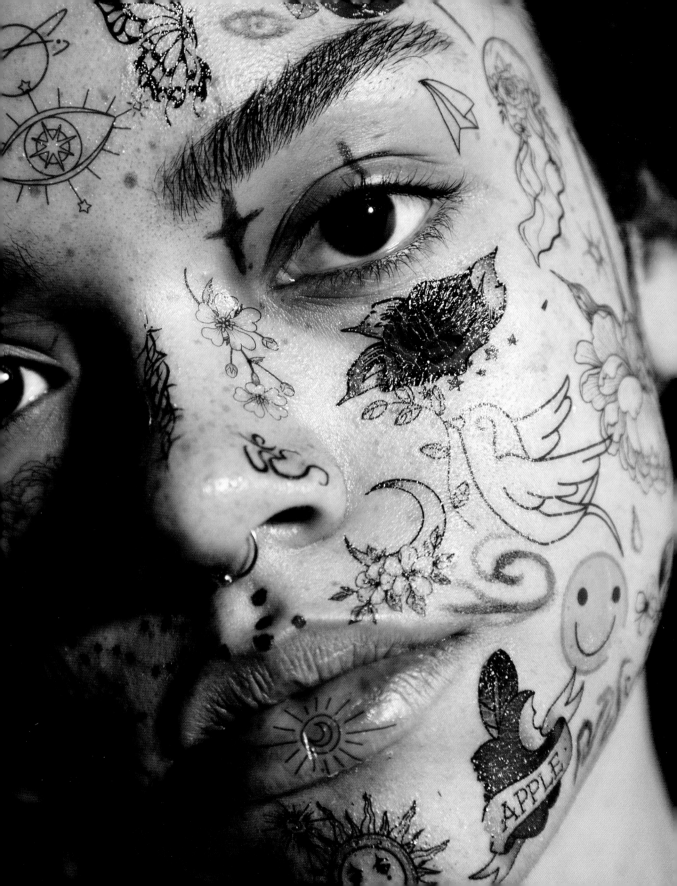

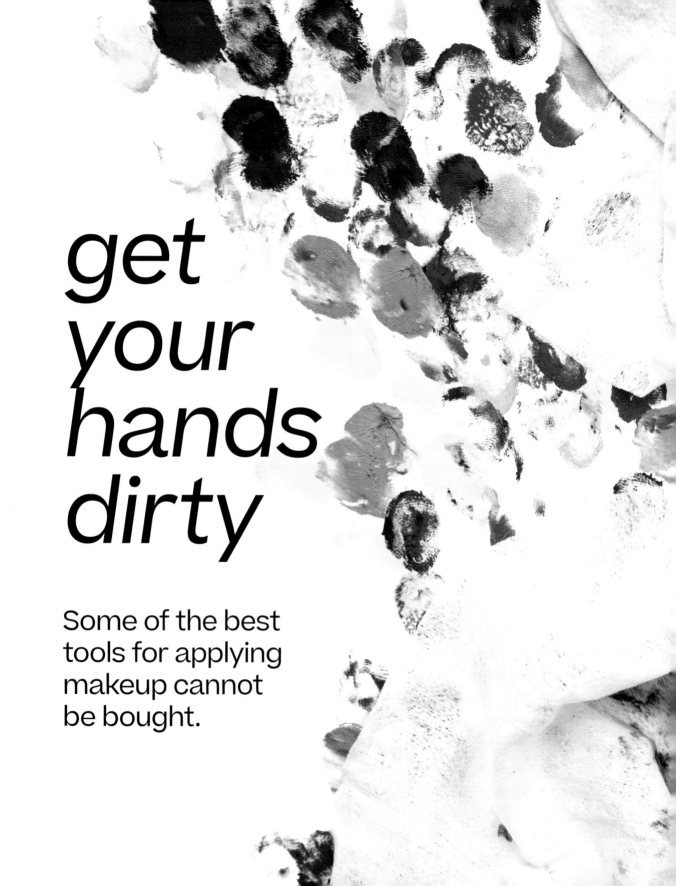

get your hands dirty

Some of the best tools for applying makeup cannot be bought.

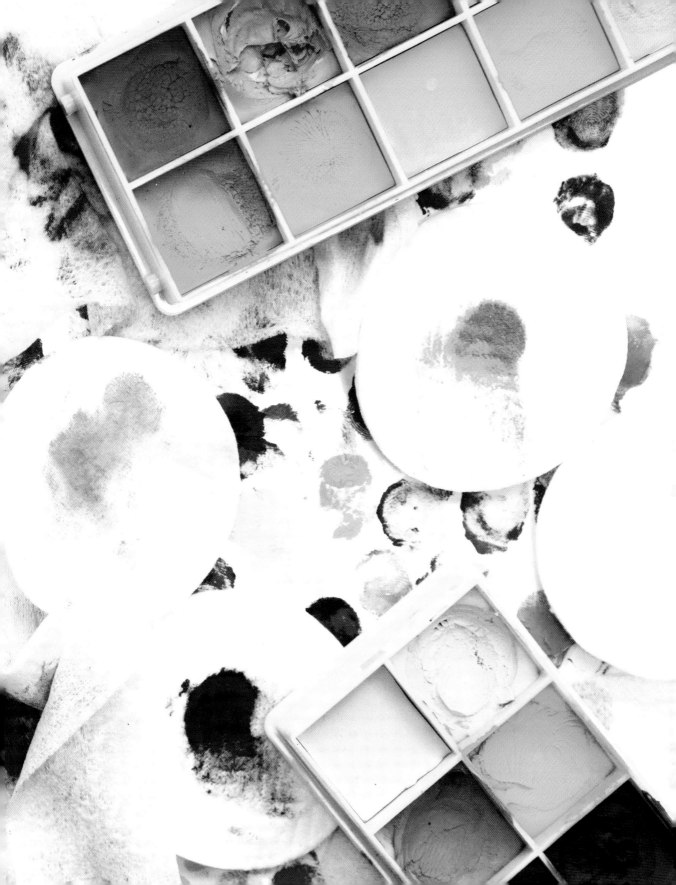

I use my fingers a lot when applying makeup. Fingers, thumbs and even the palm of your hand can be great applicators. Using a fingertip to sweep under eyeliner to extend it out, or to smudge eyeshadow or tap on a lipstick is nothing new, and it can sometimes add a human quality that brushes or sponges don't give. I was once en route to a shoot when I realised I had left every one of my brushes at home. Thankfully I couldn't leave my fingers behind, so I was able to carry out the job (although I've never forgotten my brushes since). Sometimes makeup will go on better with a finger first, as most products contain oils and the natural body temperature of the skin helps them to stick and blend by melting and softening down. The rise of swatch videos on social media has also led a move towards slightly oilier makeup, because if a product does not swatch well in a satisfying short-form video, then it might not sell.

With this experiment, you must leave your brushes behind: you are only allowed to use fingers and hands. Smudge colours with your palms, fingerpaint around the eyes, and use thumbs to apply lip stain. This doesn't need to look finessed; you are not trying to achieve the kind of precision you'd get with brushes and sponges, it's about getting up close with the product, enjoying the immediacy of blending and seeing what works on the contours of the face.

DOM SAYS

AFTER APPLYING MAKEUP WITH YOUR HANDS, USE A CLEAN FINGER TO TIDY UP ANY EDGES OR SMUDGES FOR A NEATER FINISH.

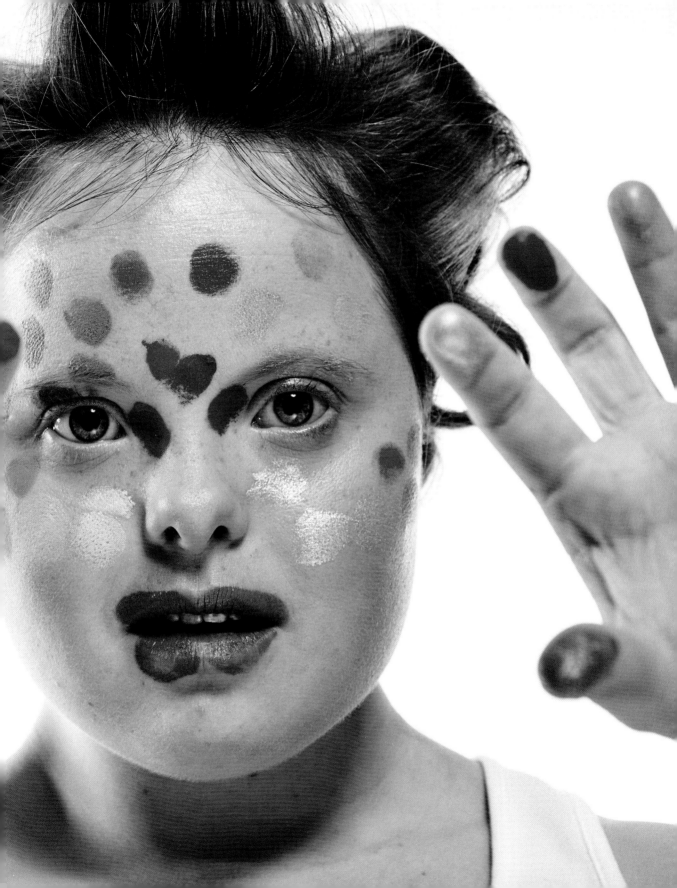

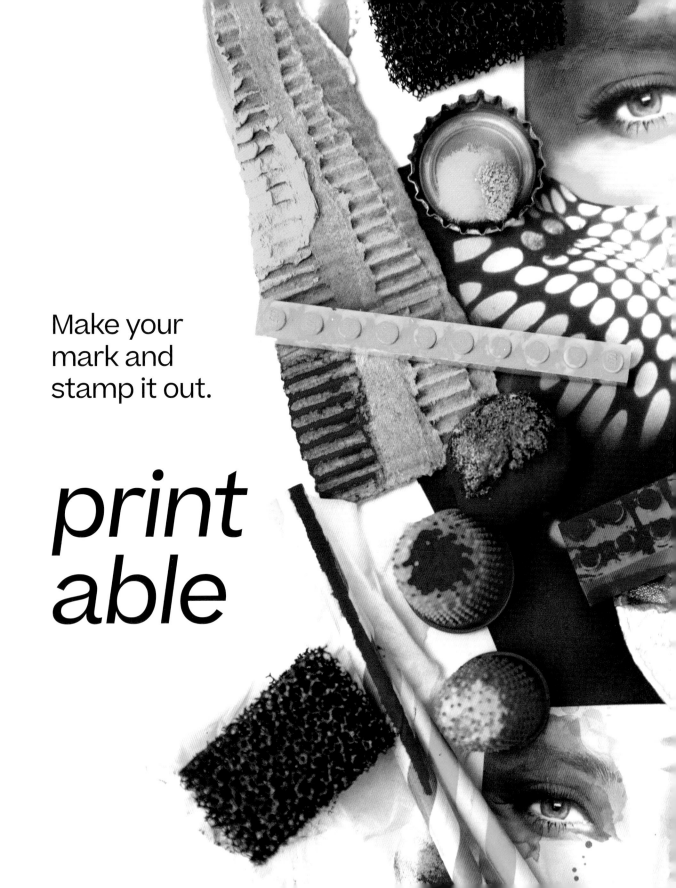

Make your
mark and
stamp it out.

*print
able*

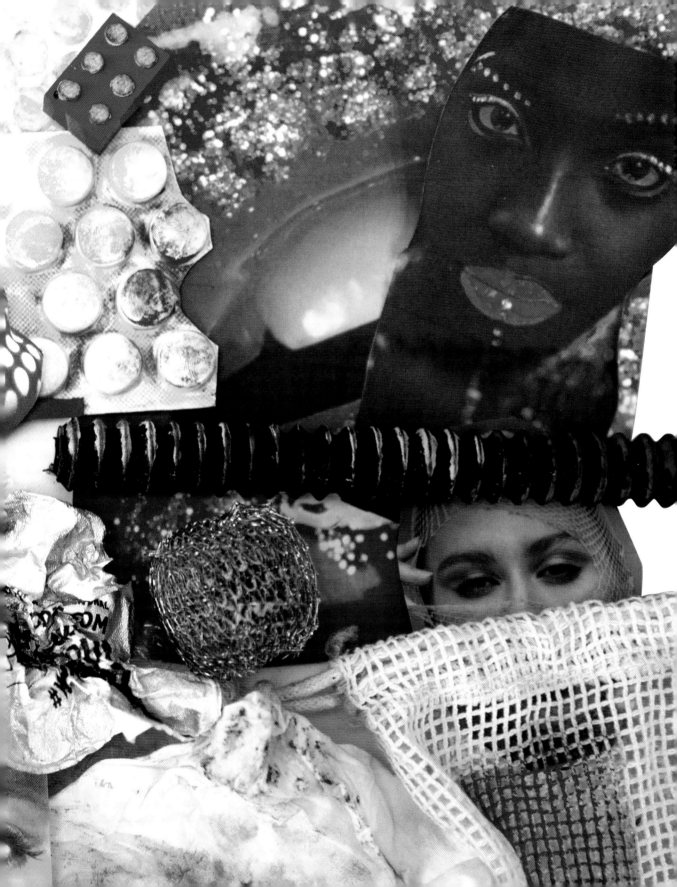

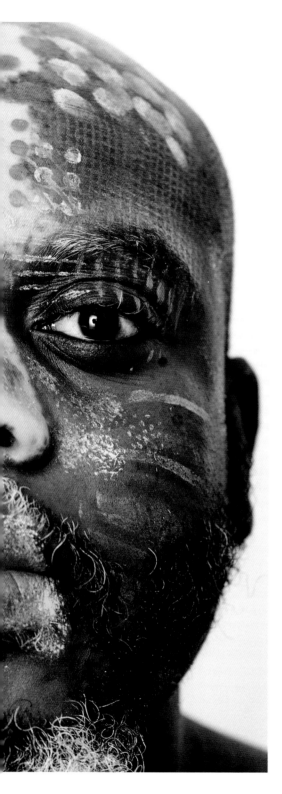

Printing onto the face can be a lot of fun, and finding things to utilise can be even more fun. I keep a stash of odd bits and bobs, things I've picked up when out and about. I try to look beyond their intended use and think about what else I can do with them. How can I repurpose this? Can I cut it? Stick it? Twist it? Smear it? Print it? Some of the most exciting makeup looks I've created have been when I added an unconventional or misplaced element: a smudge of blue over a perfect red lip; paint swept over super-clean skin with a feather. How does it look when you put a curly hair tie in black paint then roll it over a beautifully applied smoky eye? Or press bubble wrap into highlighter before stamping it onto your cheek? Try painting a Lego brick in a bright colour and pressing it over a stunning 1950s-style eyeliner. Have a go at potato printing!

I'd like you to walk through your home and collect together as many different items as you can that you think could make interesting prints on the face. After applying a simple makeup using conventional colours and techniques, embellish the look with all of the different printable objects.

DOM SAYS

WHEN PRINTING ONTO THE SKIN, LESS PRODUCT IS MORE. IF YOU OVERLOAD AN OBJECT WITH PAINT, THEN IT MIGHT MOVE AROUND TOO MUCH WHEN YOU STAMP IT. THE THINNER THE LAYER OF PAINT, THE MORE DETAIL YOU WILL ACHIEVE.

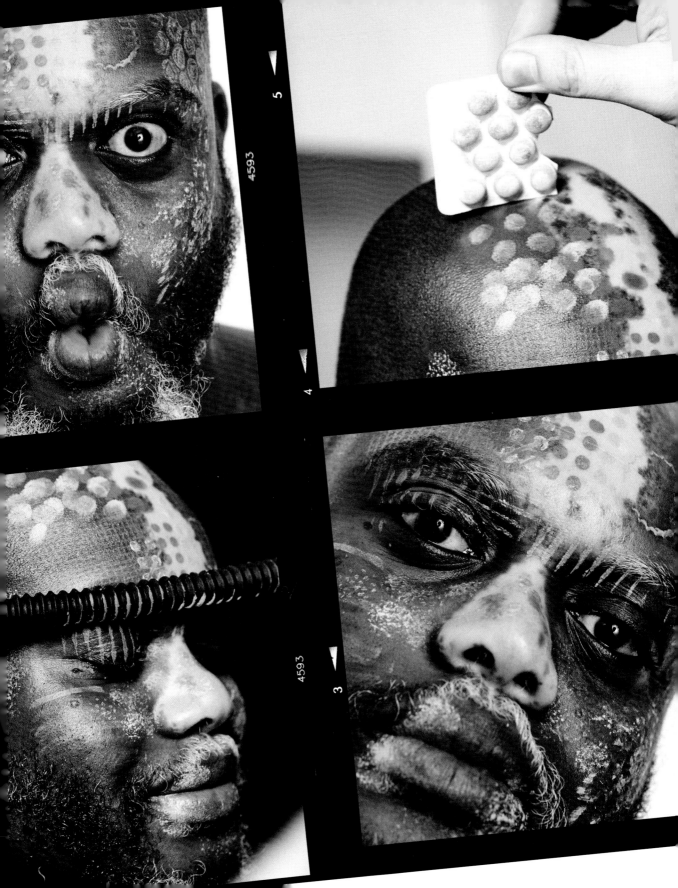

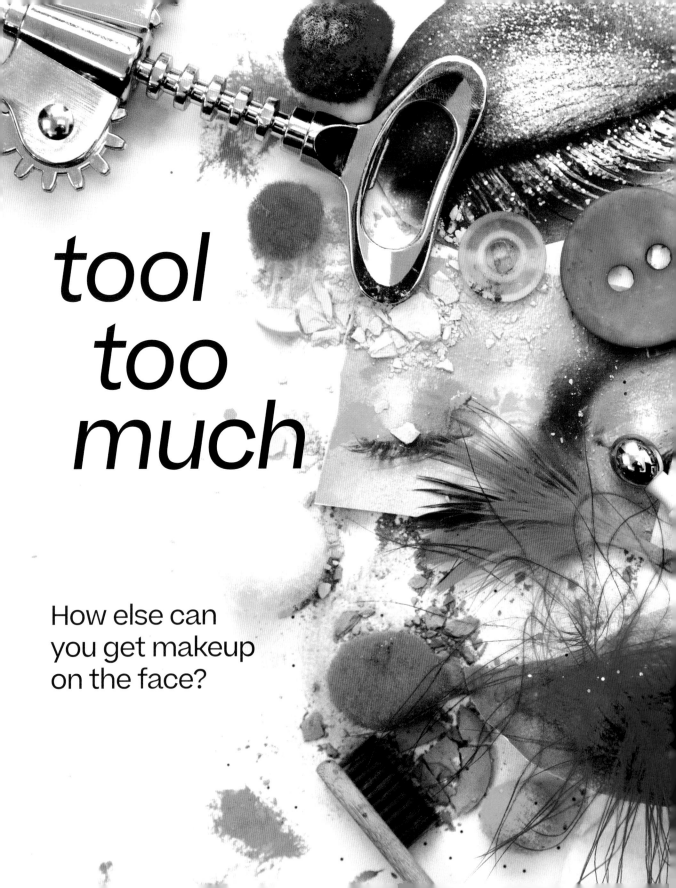

tool too much

How else can you get makeup on the face?

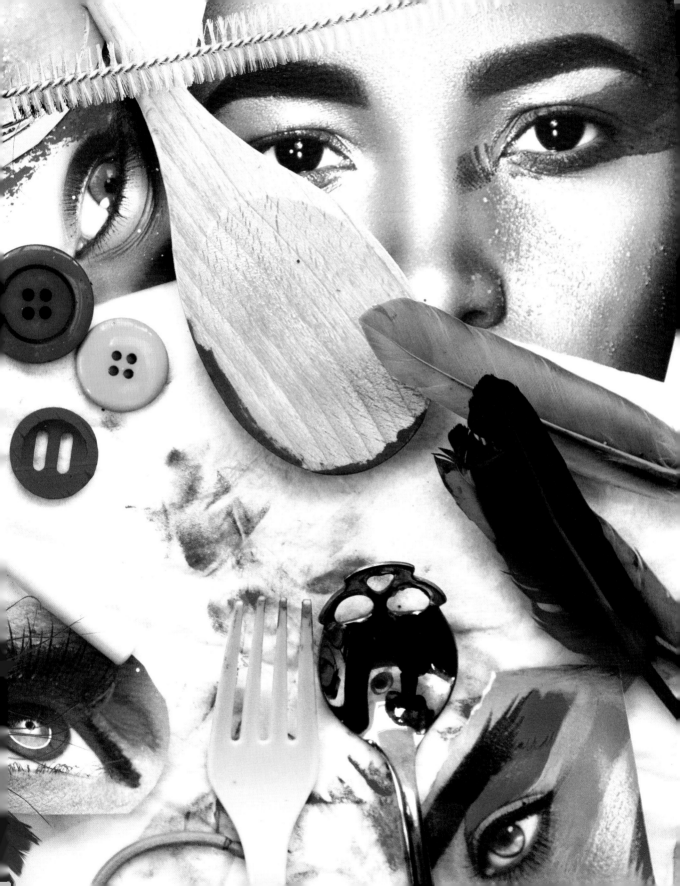

The world is your oyster... it could even be an oyster.

What is a makeup brush? It's a tool, something that functions to get makeup on the face. Each type of brush has been specially designed to deliver product in different ways to enable artists to create more easily whatever effect they're after. However, relying on brushes can limit the creative process and anchor you in the convention of traditional makeup. But pretty much anything can be used as a tool, to help unlock imaginative potential.

Have a look around, and see what might deliver a unique application. Instead of using a conventional brush to apply eyeshadow, how about lightly scrunching up some tissue, pressing it onto the eyeshadow and rolling it over the eye? Or drip the end of a shoelace in liquid eyeliner and drag it across the eyelid? Could you make a repeat dot design using a cotton swab? Maybe cover string in a liquid or cream product and roll it back and forth over the cheek? The round eraser on the end of a pencil could fit the lip shape rather well to dab on a lip stain. The opportunities are endless. Could you use the back of a spoon? A button? A feather? An old necklace? These alternative tools can take quite ordinary applications and give them a fresh vibe. The world is your oyster... you might even use an oyster!

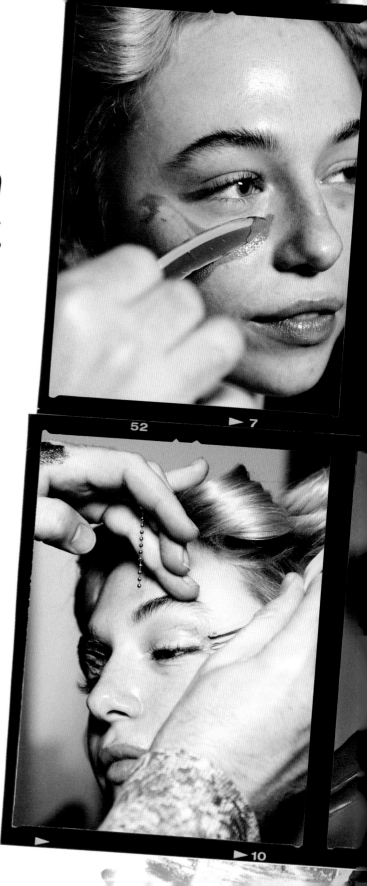

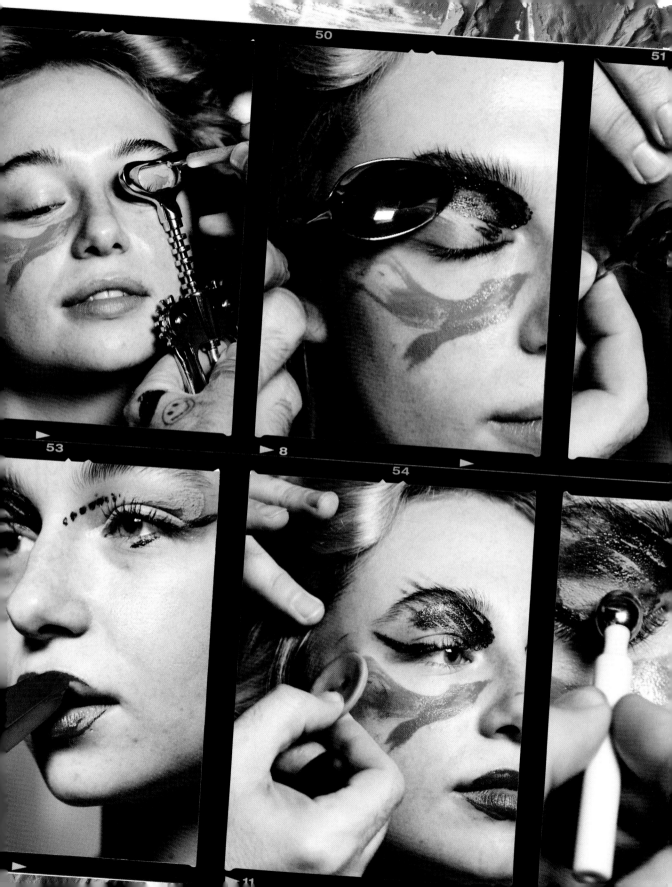

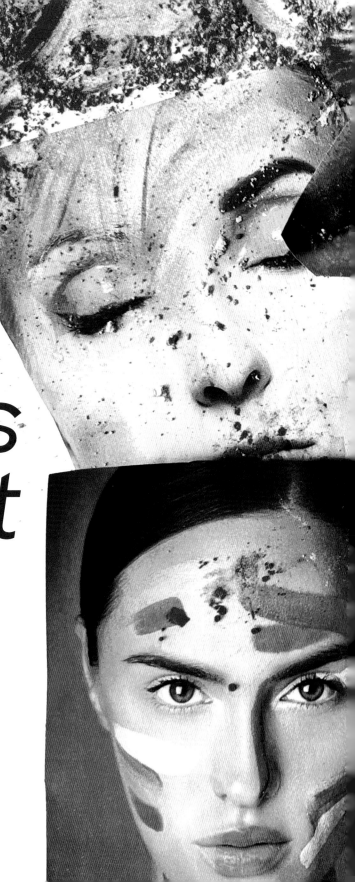

oppo sites attract

Get versatile
and switch
up your left
and right.

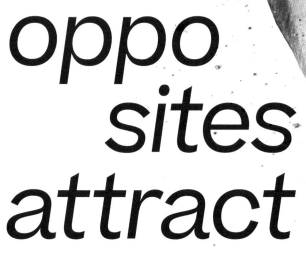

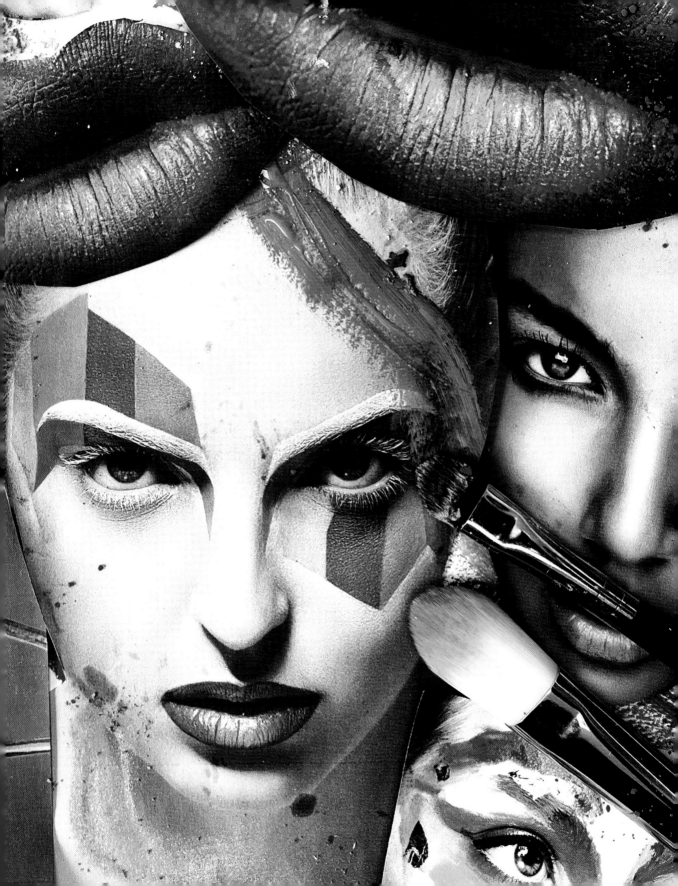

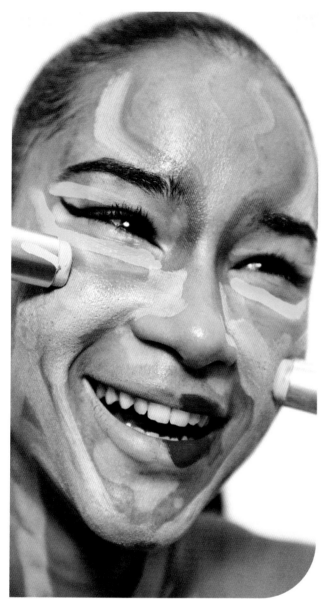

I've always been fascinated by people who are ambidextrous, especially artists. To have creativity flow from both your left and right hands is amazing. Sadly I do not share this ability, but over the years I have forced myself to use my left hand at times so I'm not so reliant on my right. As a makeup artist this is a tremendous skill to have. Firstly, the simple act of using one hand for the left eye and that same hand for the right doesn't really make sense: the hand has to move in two different directions to try to create symmetry. Surely it would be more logical for each hand to do the same action for better precision. Secondly, MUA's often just don't have much space to move around. When using only your left or right hand, you must get yourself into different, often awkward, positions around the model to achieve the correct angles.

I have trained myself to be able to pass the brush from right to left, and that's what this exercise gets you to practise. Apply a look using your right hand to make up the right side of the face, and your left hand to make up the left side. I'm not going to say it's not challenging, but it can also be really fun. Using your opposite hand can be super freeing: our muscle memory sometimes means we don't need to think about what we are doing, so this brings us back to the moment.

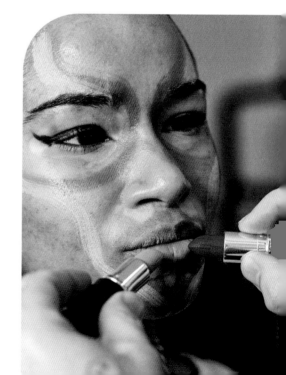

Play into the wibbles. Use them to create interesting lines and shapes.

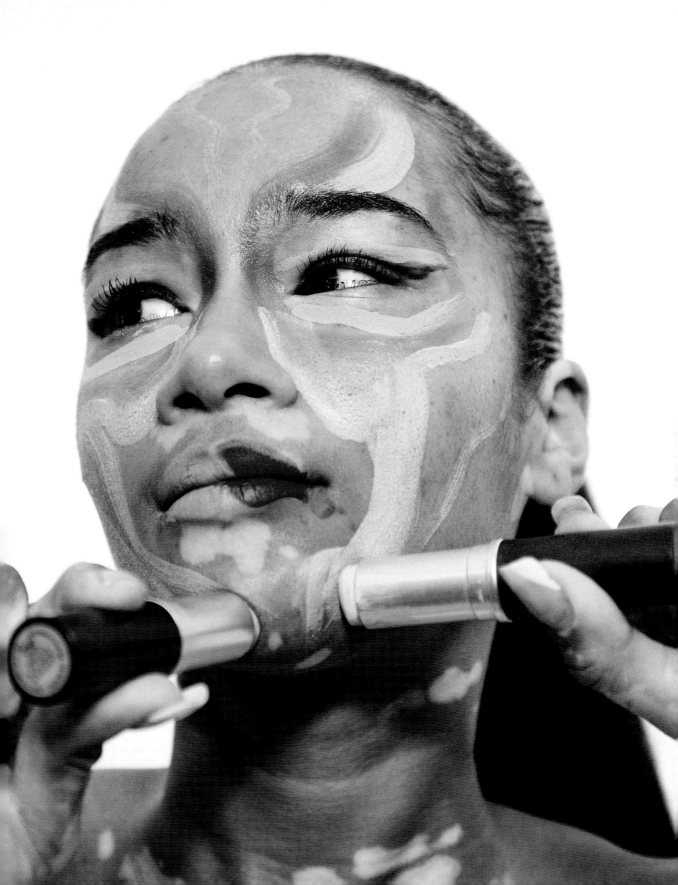

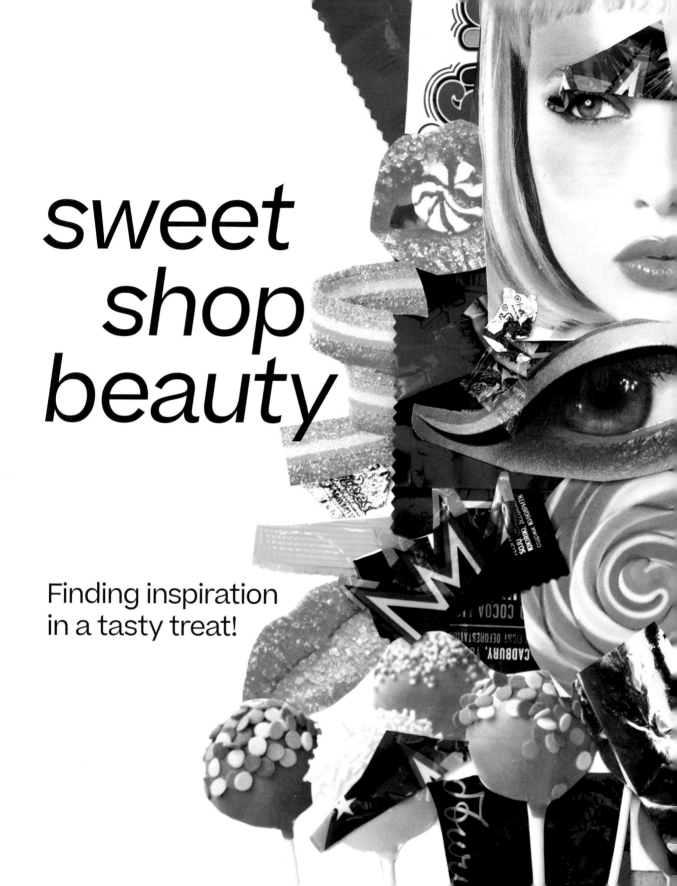

sweet shop beauty

Finding inspiration
in a tasty treat!

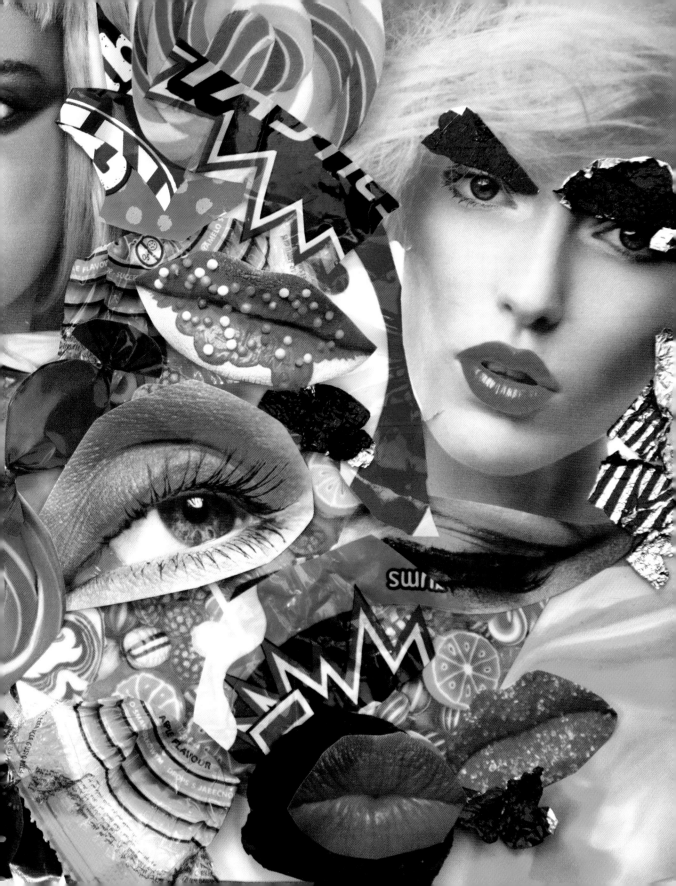

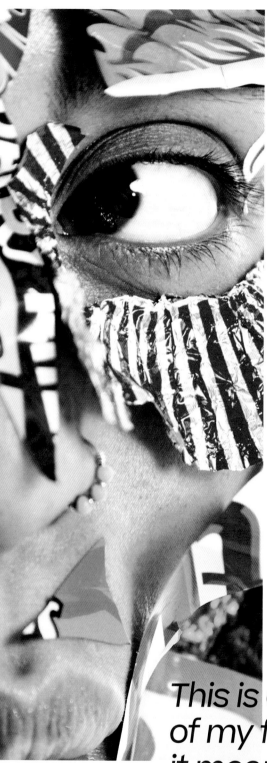

DOM SAYS

DON'T EAT THE CANDY STRAIGHT
AFTER PUTTING ON YOUR MAKEUP
IF YOU'RE INCORPORATING A
STRONG LIP, IT MIGHT SMUDGE!
BEST TO EAT IT WHILE WORKING
THROUGH YOUR LOOK.

Colour theory isn't too hard to get your head
around. It is used everywhere and especially in
advertising, particularly when the advert needs
to fight for your attention. Take items in a sweet
shop. They all burst with colour so you buy them.
How do they stand out so much? Well, it's down
to colour theory. Opposites attract. If you use
two colours directly across from each other in
the colour wheel (known as complementary
colours), like red and green or yellow and purple,
the colours will look like they are pulsating or
vibrating. Another aspect of colour theory is
triadic colour: the power of three, which refers
to three evenly spaced colours like red/yellow/
blue or green/purple/orange. Sometimes these
two colour groupings 'marry' and create 'split
complimentaries', where you take one colour,
orange, say, and instead of pairing it with the
colour opposite (blue), you pair it with the two
colours next to its opposite: green or purple.
      These colour group concepts, used all the
time in confectionary, are a great way of helping
you use unconventional or unusual colours in
your makeup. Buy a variety of sweets and
chocolate bars. Close your eyes and rummage
through the treats. Whichever one you pull out is
not only the one you get to eat but the colours
on the wrapper are the colours you must use in
you makeup, not in a total recreation but using
the flow and patterns on the wrapper. Maybe
scrunch the wrapper and recreate what you see.

This is experiment is one of my favourites because it means eating sweets!

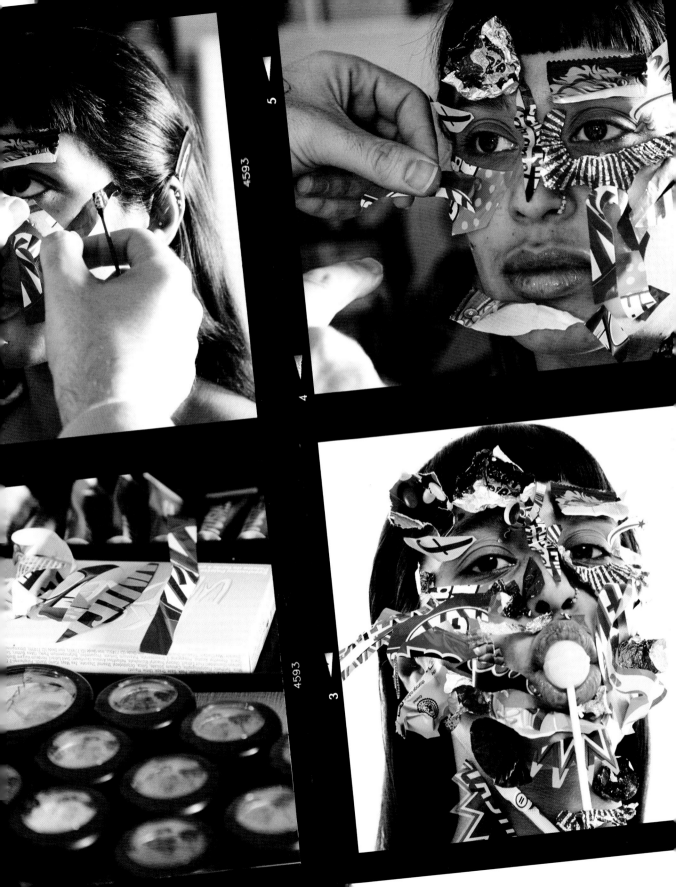

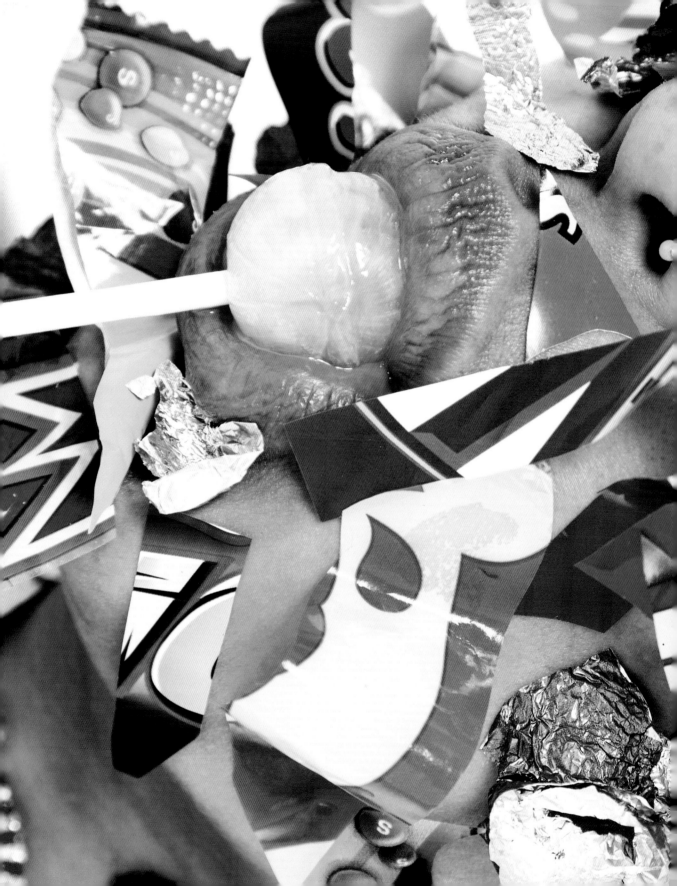

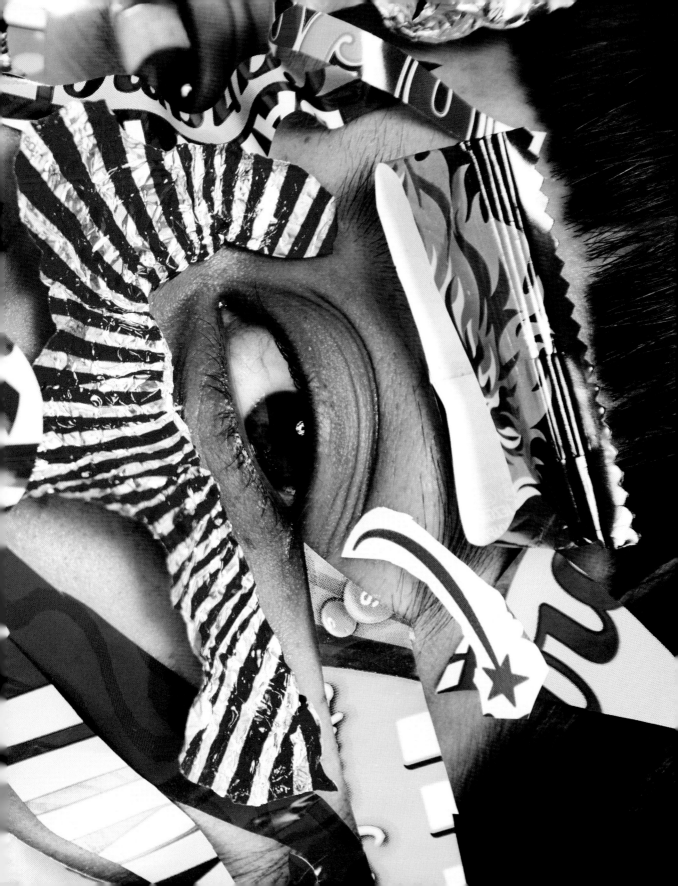

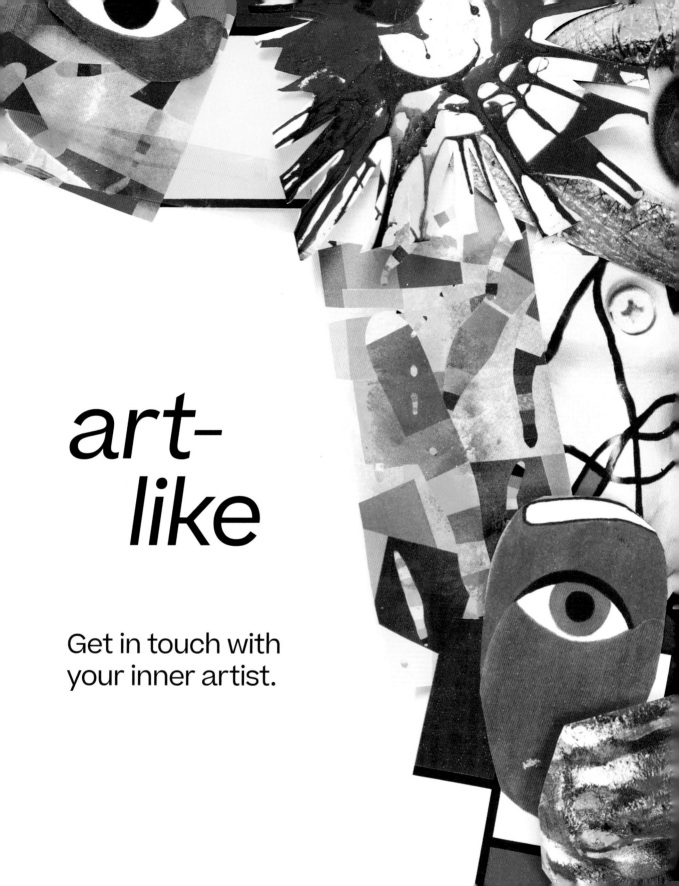

art-
like

Get in touch with
your inner artist.

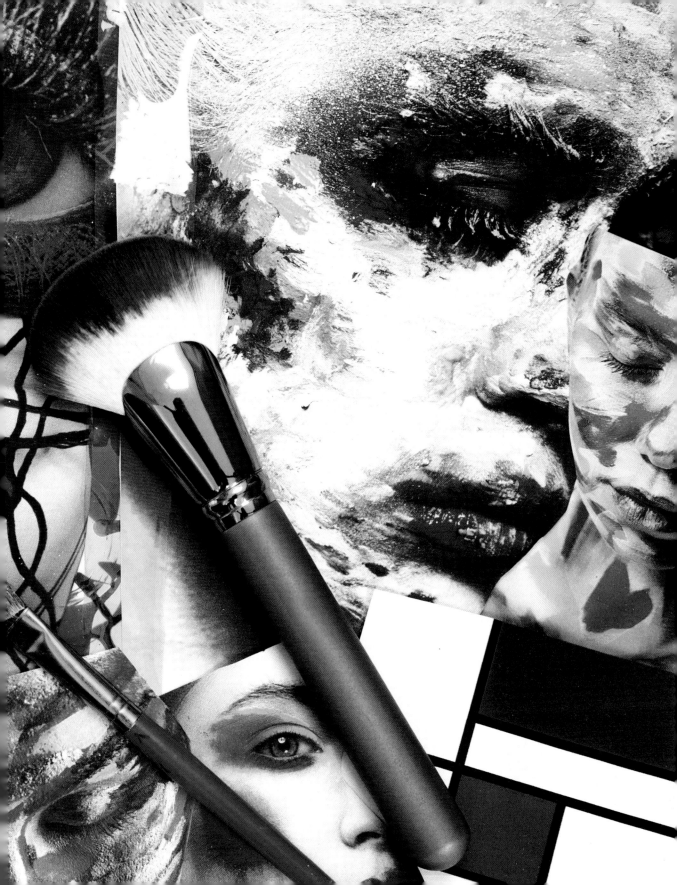

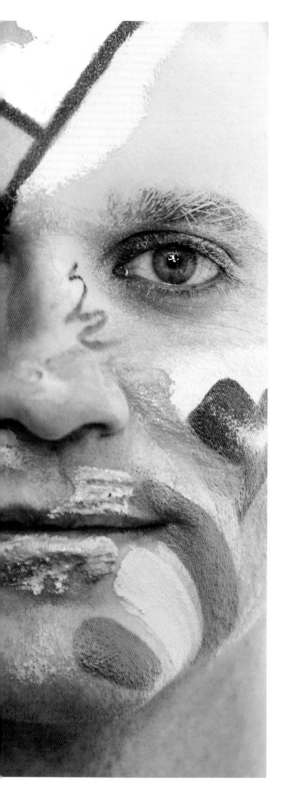

This challenge is about thinking like a painter.

All makeup artists are painters at heart. It's important to feed the soul with artistic inspiration to help connect you to different mediums and styles, which you can then bring to your work. Choose a favourite painting, artist or movement and use it as a springboard to create your makeup: perhaps you're drawn to the crazy geometry of Picasso, the colourful chaos of Jackson Pollock's unbridled abstraction, or the soft-focus blur of Monet.

    This challenge is not about how good at drawing you are, it's about thinking like a painter and seeing the world in new ways. Consider how you might translate key features from a painting or art movement, or interpret an artist's signature style through makeup. Be enthused by the bold colours of Pop Art; experiment with dreamy Surrealist swirls; layer on product to create a textured Expressionistic masterpiece; apply tiny dots of pure colour to emulate the eye-fooling techniques of Pointillism; create seamless colour blends to evoke the Impressionists. Focus on texture, colour and technique, particularly brushwork, to create your makeup masterpiece

DOM SAYS

DON'T BE AFRAID TO ADD UNIQUE TOUCHES TO CAPTURE THE ESSENCE OF YOUR CHOSEN ARTIST OR STYLE. THIS COULD BE FACIAL DECALS, OR EVEN PAINTING SMALL MOTIFS SUCH AS HEARTS AND CLOUDS THAT EVOKE PARTICULAR ARTWORKS.

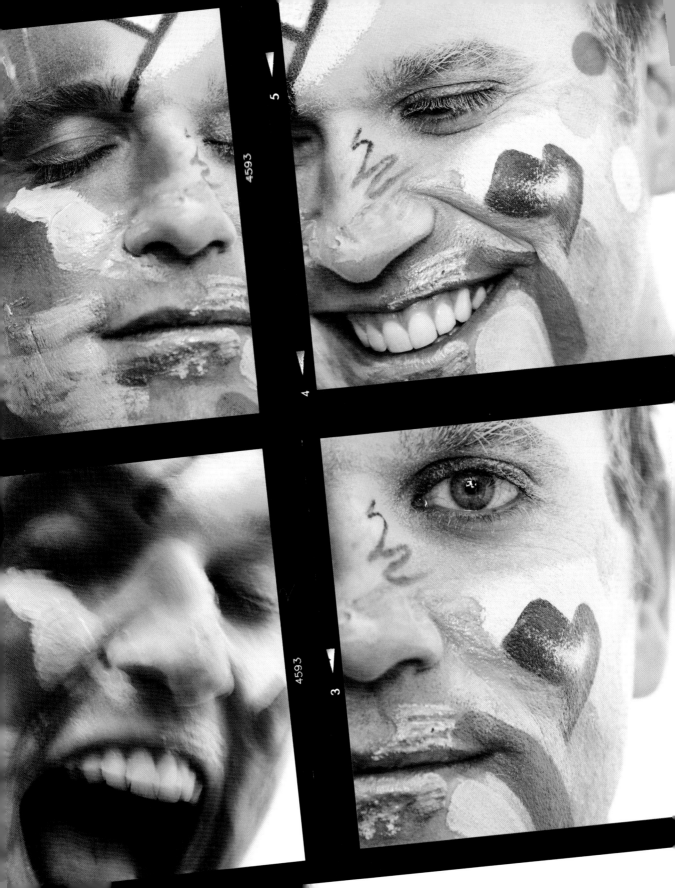

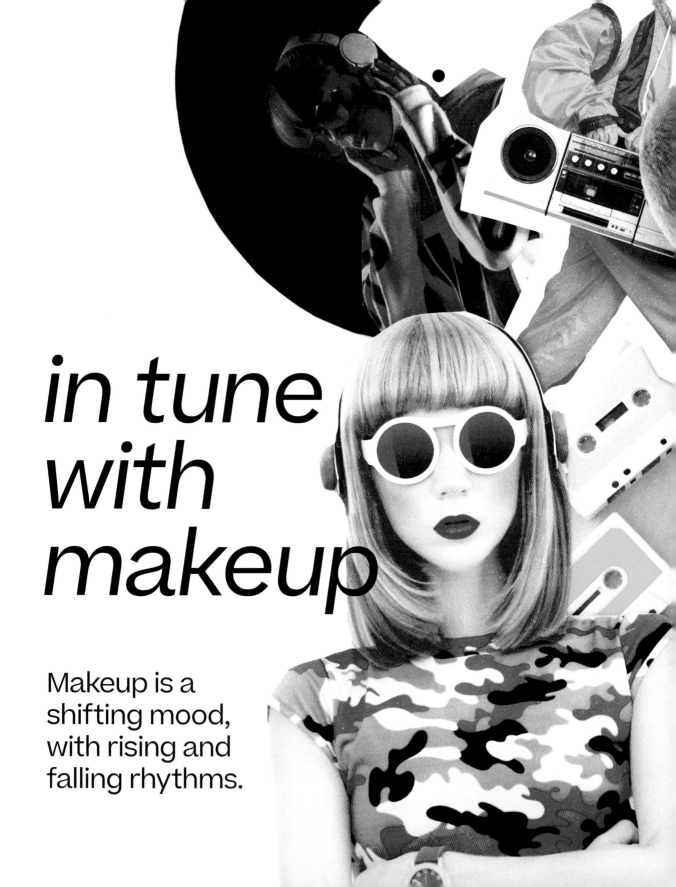

in tune with makeup

Makeup is a shifting mood, with rising and falling rhythms.

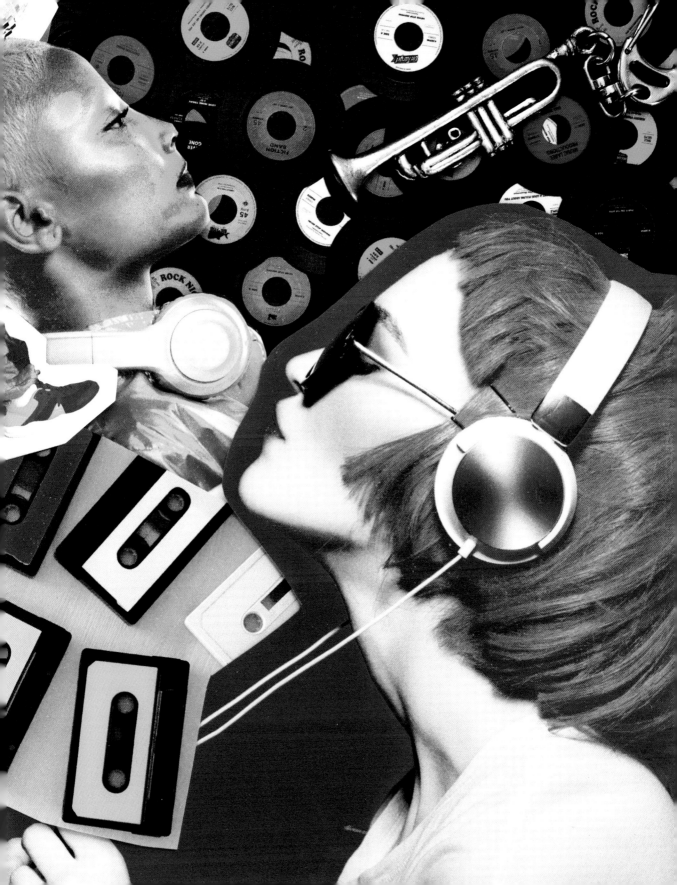

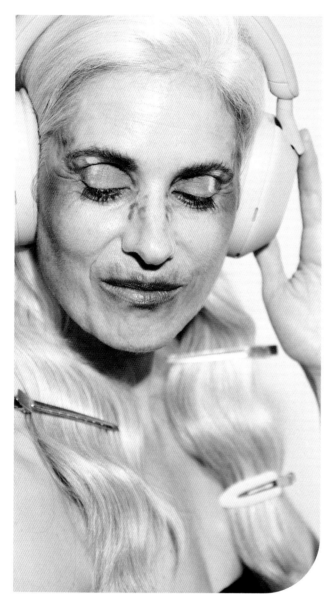

Who doesn't play music when getting ready to go out? It's like having a hype man, pumping us up into a frenzy; it sets the tone and helps get us in the mood. The energy from the music transfers into how we dress, how we move, and how we do our makeup. When you're an MUA working with recording artists, really getting their vibe is vital. Each artist is unique, and a way to access their spirit is through really listening to their music and disconnecting from what's going on around, feeling your way into the mood. Sure, the artist has their established style, but the makeup you create can play a vital role in building that narrative.

With this music-inspired experiment, you can practise using music to shut off the mundane world and transport yourself into an imaginative space. Start by shuffling your playlist. Close your eyes for the first few moments and just listen. As the first track progresses, start applying your makeup. As the song changes, close your eyes again and connect to the mood of the track, then continue. If a song changes mid-way through working on a feature, then consciously change the style in accordance with the feel of the tune now playing: perhaps a sulky grunge eye turns glittery when a disco banger drops, or your bubble-gum pop lip becomes a shade darker when the tempo turns more downbeat.

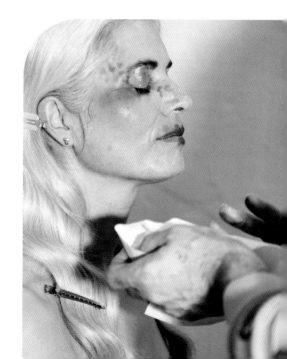

Find those happy accidents when one style of makeup may clash with another.

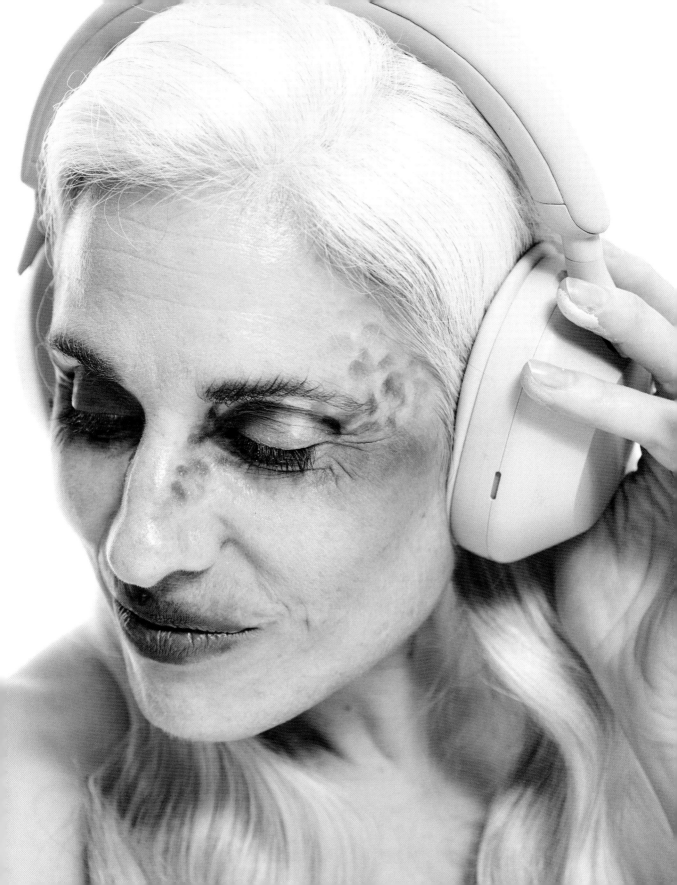

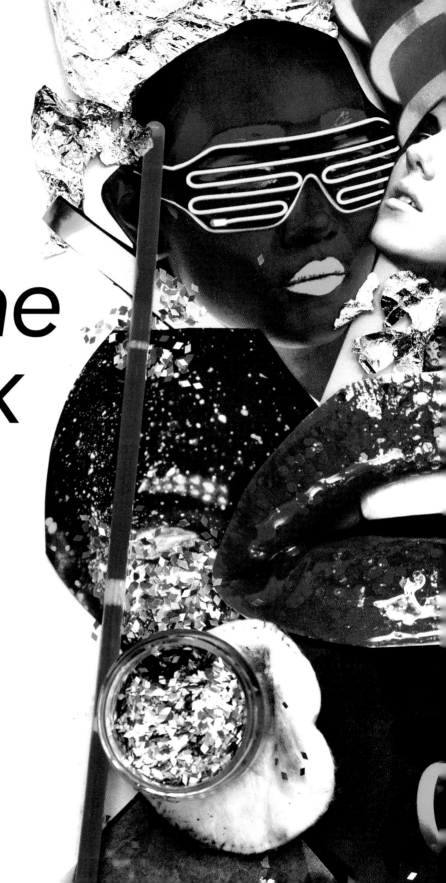

in the
dark

Beauty
blindfolded.

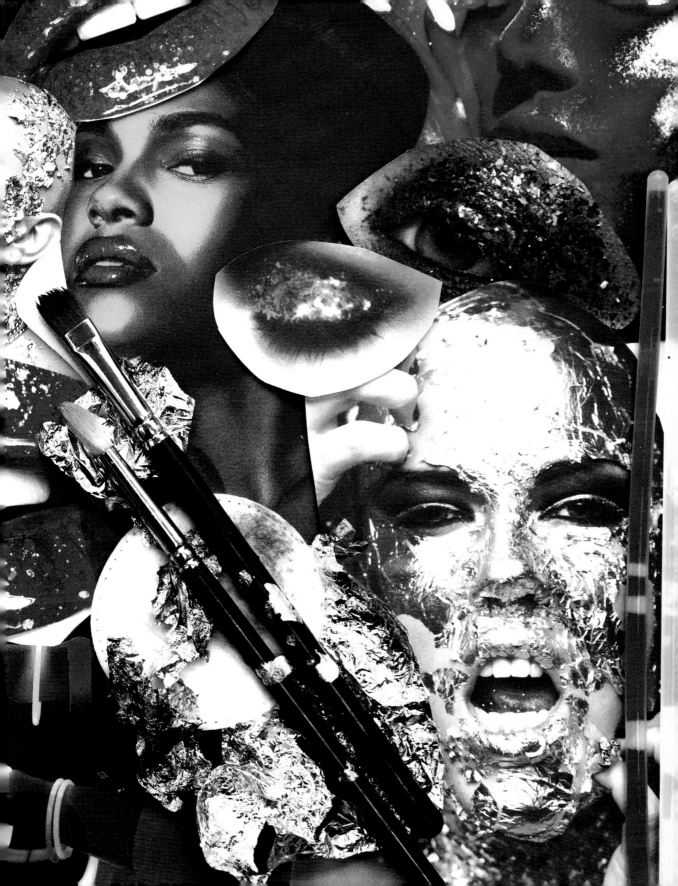

The idea is to free yourself really go for it!

The subconscious plays a huge part in our makeup choices. Our brain tricks us into thinking we have free will, but really it is always guiding us to make familiar, comfortable 'choices'. But where's the fun in that? Where's the chaos and creativity? For this experiment you will need to blindfold yourself if you're working on someone else, or find a room with no windows and turn off the lights if you are working on your own face. Prep your area by laying out your makeup so you know roughly where things are, but try not to memorise this too precisely. Once you're prepped, step into the dark and start your makeup application.

The purpose of this challenge is to surrender your control over the products and colours you are using. The idea is to free yourself from the confines of subconscious thought and just go for it. Once you've applied the makeup, take your blindfold off and see what you have produced. It's not necessarily going to be pretty, but that's the point. It's about seeing what shouldn't work but actually maybe does. This will help you see colour relationships differently, and discover how imprecise application can actually look great. You might be surprised by how fresh the results seem.

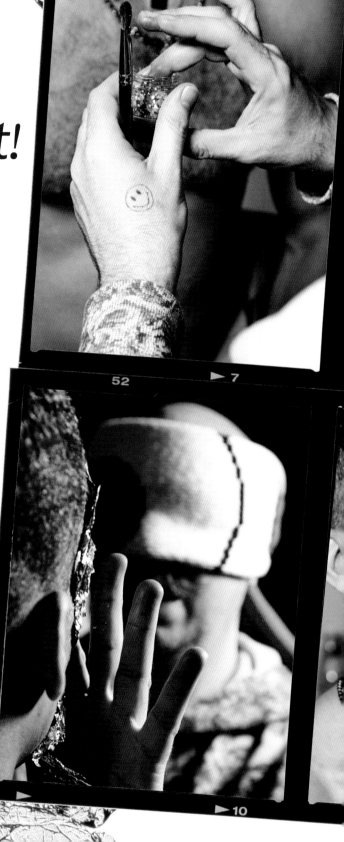

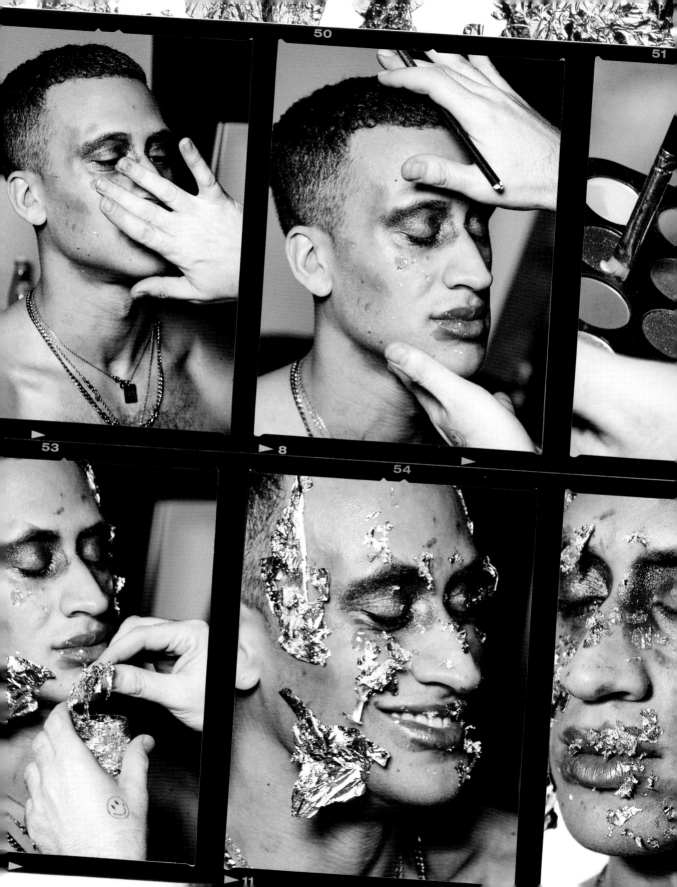

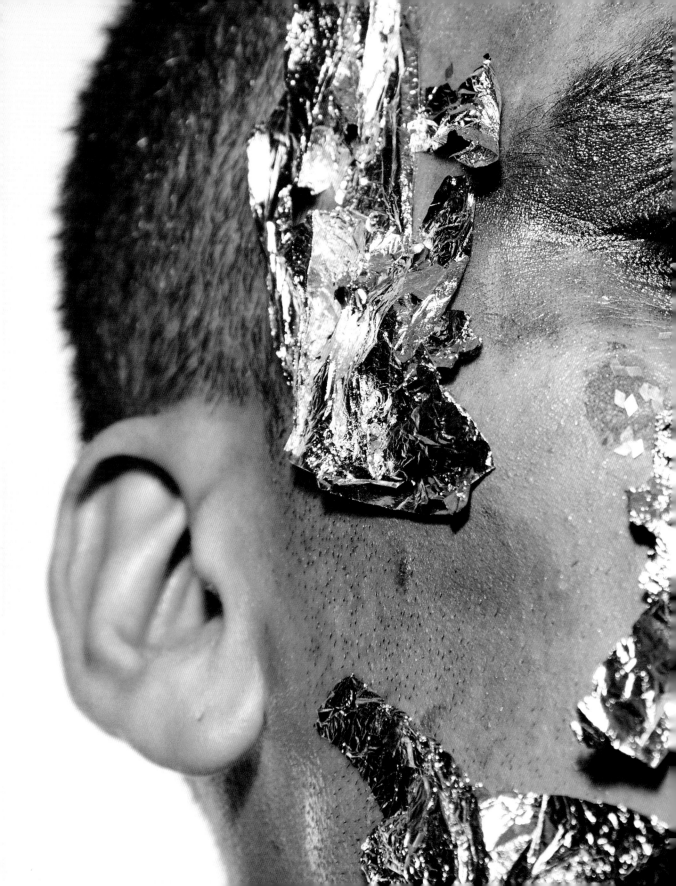

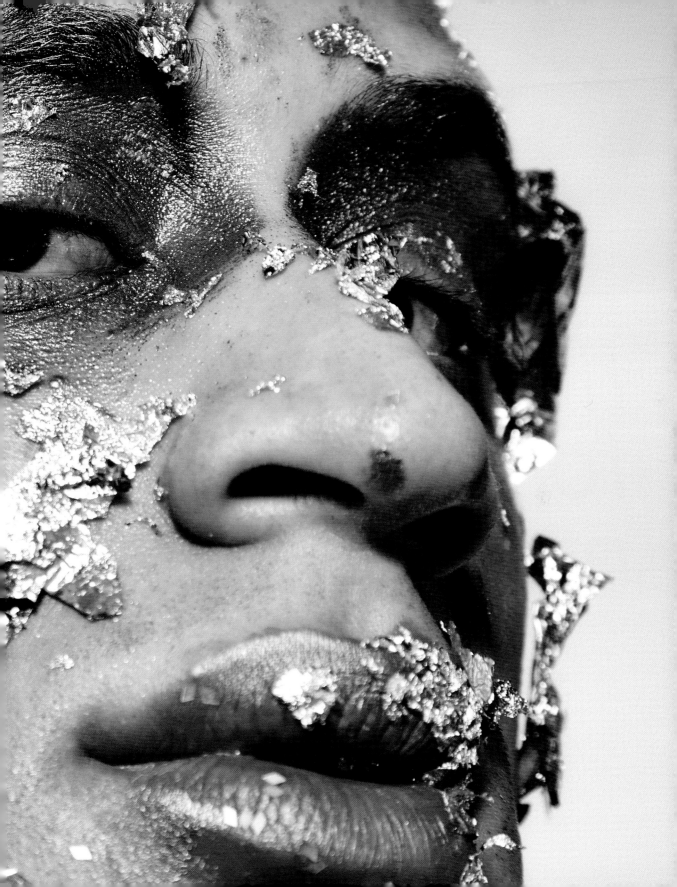

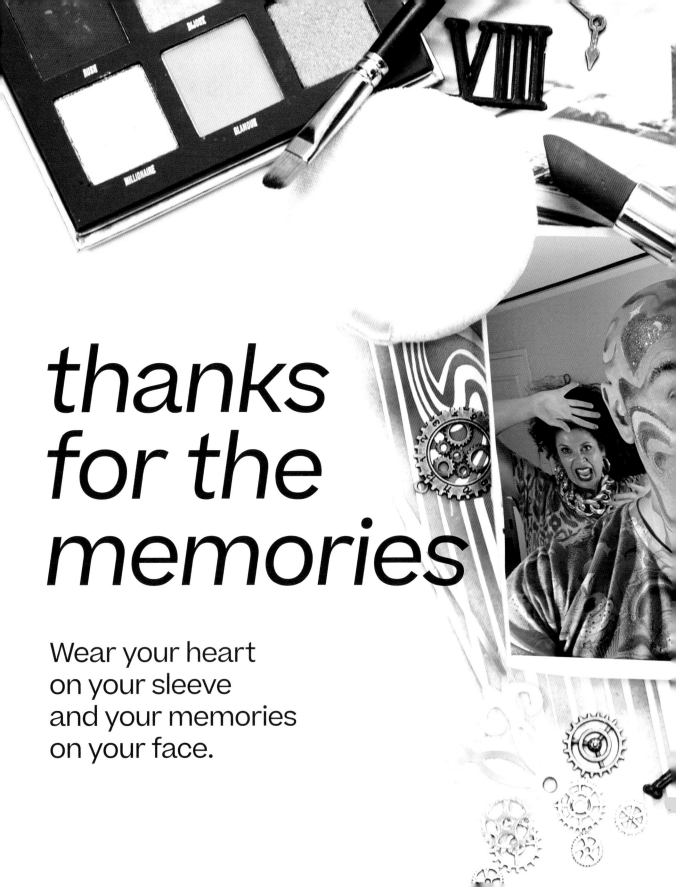

thanks for the memories

Wear your heart
on your sleeve
and your memories
on your face.

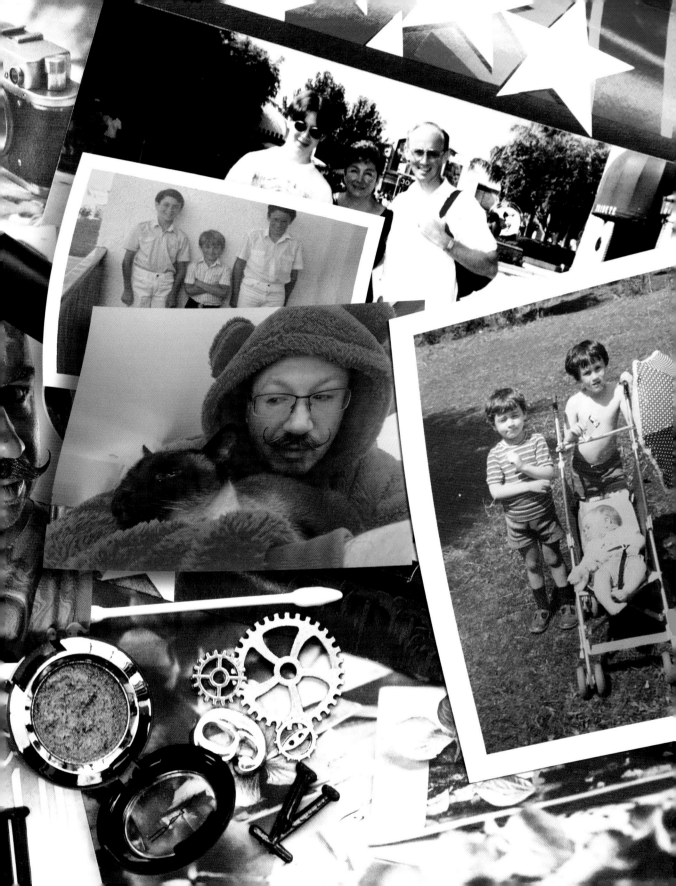

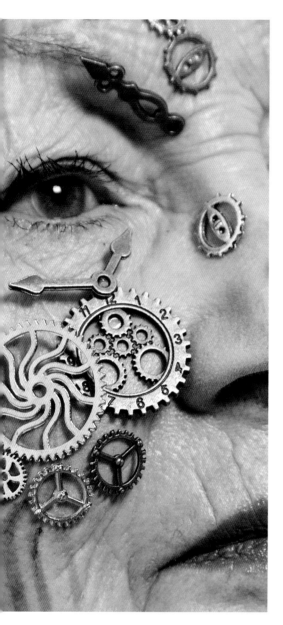

Finding inspiration in the world around us is relatively easy, you just need to look. We've experimented with various ways of finding inspiration from life, from influential artists (p.82) to favourite sweets (p.76). We are surrounded by so many different things that we can look to for ideas: the design on a coffee cup, the texture of a table, even the random colours of pens in a pot, but what do these objects mean to us? By exploring mood via music (p.86), we were able to tap into mindfulness and connect our makeup to the emotions we felt when we heard certain songs. Now we will look at how visuals evoke feelings by finding inspiration in something that is meaningful to us.

Look around for something that elicits a strong memory: it could be a photo from a great holiday with friends, something that someone you love bought for you, or was left to you by a loved one. Whatever the object is, really think about how it makes you feel. Use it to tap into deep emotion to create your next makeup look. Try to match feelings up with colours, and consider how you could relay the textures and shapes of the object in your makeup.

Carrying the meaningful object around with you in the form of your makeup is a wonderful way to keep that memory close.

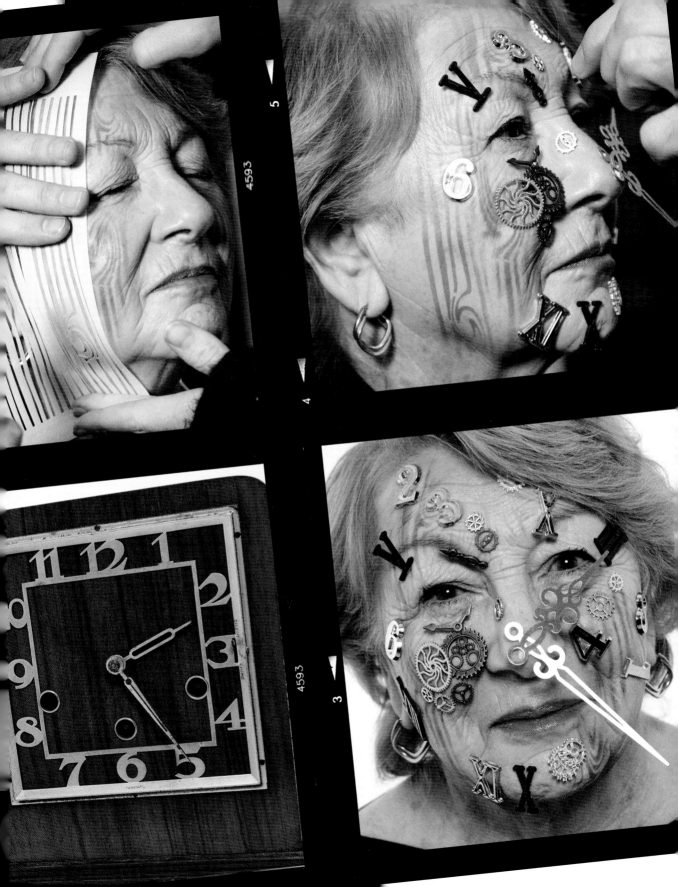

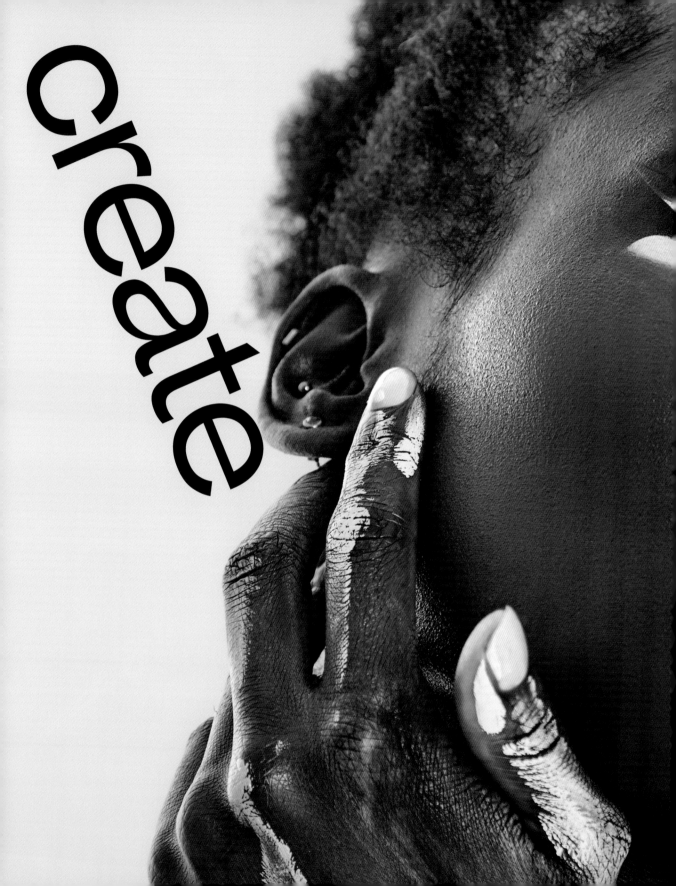

create

2

the

look

Now that you've had fun daubing your fingers in things, raiding the kitchen cabinets, playing at racing cars, looking at ordinary objects anew and getting messy with makeup, it's time to examine the results. Here you'll look at the images you captured during the experiments and search for those hidden moments of glory that you can expand and build upon to create a finessed makeup look. I have loved taking what I discovered and developing the full makeup looks within this chapter.

It's worth taking your time to look at all aspects of what you have created at the experimental stage: there may be a great colour combination, but perhaps in the wrong place; there could be a detail positioned in an interesting way, but the colour doesn't necessarily work; maybe a successful layering of things that shouldn't really go together. The key is to zoom in and really look, examining every part of the experiment.

Once you have an idea of how you're going to elaborate on a happy accident, consider how bold you want to go. Learning when to edit and when not to hold back is a skill that can take a long time to master. You don't need to throw everything at each look, but it can be really fun to go big. Try starting with a simple application and then build, capturing images at each step, until you've taken it too far. This will enable you to look back at what you've created and see where the balance was before it tipped into crazy. This tipping point is different for everyone, but by playing around you'll begin to figure what yours is.

In the previous chapter you saw where I went with each experiment, and now you'll discover what parts I developed into a final look. Each of these looks in this chapter was completed straight after the experiment. Once we had photographed the experimental look, it all came off and I went straight in with the editorial look, giving myself no more than an hour to change things around before we photographed them again. This time constraint was both friend and foe: it stopped me from overthinking and made me just do it, allowing for true spontaneity, but at other times it meant I wasn't able to think things through completely. But this book is not about me and what I can do. It's about you. Seeing what someone else does certainly helps, but it's about getting a sense of what's possible and how a brief might be interpreted. So rather than trying to follow exactly what I did, look at how I developed the results of my experiments into a concept for a look to help you work out how to develop yours.

While there are images that I love in this chapter, the real interest for me lies in the continuing process. How might these creative looks develop next? How would they move on? Could some be combined? Or are there two ideas within one look that need separating out? Remember, you're on a journey to find your own unique take and style – there's no fun in racing to the final destination.

hot

In developing this editorial look (p.16), it all came down to the model that I had in my chair. I noticed that the cold colours made my model's brown eyes really pop, the iris intensified and almost appeared to change colour. So I decided to take this colour group and use it throughout the look. I find that temperatures within colours direct the feel and vibe of the look. As I went for a cold colour story, I felt it would be appropriate to make this look romantic. The interesting thing about colour temperature is that there is some crossover. Pink, for example, is a tint of red, a hot colour, but it can become a cool colour when a drop of blue is added. Texture can also play a role in the feel of an image. As this is a cold look, I decided to incorporate more matte products to help bring the story more depth.

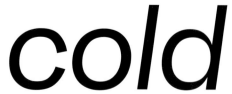

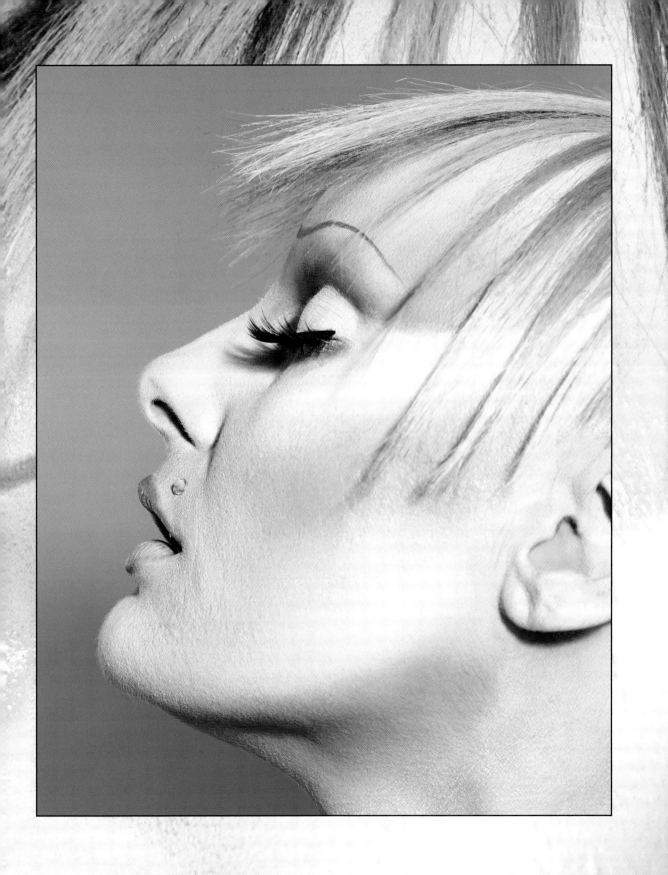

Priming the eye or applying a base help the colour to go on with impact.

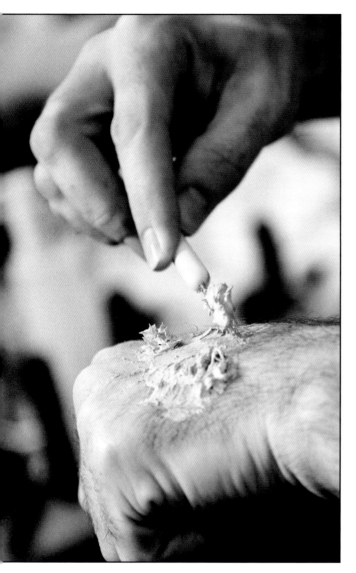

Here's how to create an editorial look based around these elements.

Using three different shades of blue (light, medium and dark), create a blue base over the whole face: the lightest shade acts as a highlighter, the darkest as a contour and the medium shade goes over the rest of the skin. Use a makeup sponge to seamlessly blend the different tones, and then set with a blue powder. Keep going until the neck and shoulders are also covered.

Apply a bright blue eyeshadow through the socket line, sweeping it out towards the temple and wrapping it around the nose to follow the orbital bone.

Intensify this with deep shades of blue in the socket and lighter shades on the eyelid.

Use a deep blue pencil to line the lips before filling them with lighter blue using a flat brush. Finish with some gloss over top.

To draw the eyebrows, wet a very fine brush and work it into some deep blue shadow, starting slightly above the brow line and following the natural shape of the brow – add a subtle up-tick at the start to give character.

Mark the placement for the jewel with a white pencil, then use a cotton swab and lash glue to precisely adhere the blue gem to the face.

Attach some false lashes, then apply mascara to both the false and real lashes to blend them together.

Priming can also help prevent any staining when using stronger or intense colours.

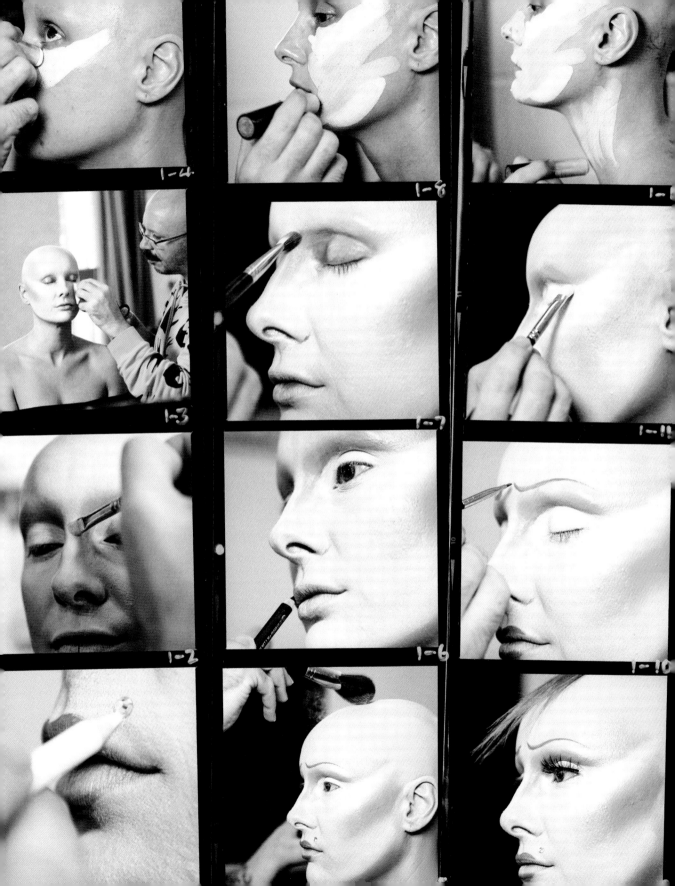

mono

The idea of using just one colour is nothing new, and colour blocking is a classic technique in design and art, but it can be a refreshing way to limit your options and so force you into a new way of thinking about makeup. Sometimes limitations can be our best asset when trying to harness creativity. And I knew that with this model I wanted to create something extraordinary. Using only one colour but in multiple products can be subtle and beautiful, but it can easily turn into something quite flat and boring – and my model was anything but. I really liked how the experiment (p.20) led me to play with pressure. Applying greater pressure gave an intense depth of hue, whereas a more delicate touch lent a lightness to the finish and subtlety to the colour. I wanted to explore this further, and look at light and heavy applications as well as positive and negative space. Why apply a colour to the eyelid when you could use it everywhere but the lid? Why apply product to the lip when you can go further than the lip? Applying a single colour to unconventional parts of the face and body can create real interest, taking the makeup beyond the norm to become something otherworldly.

chrome

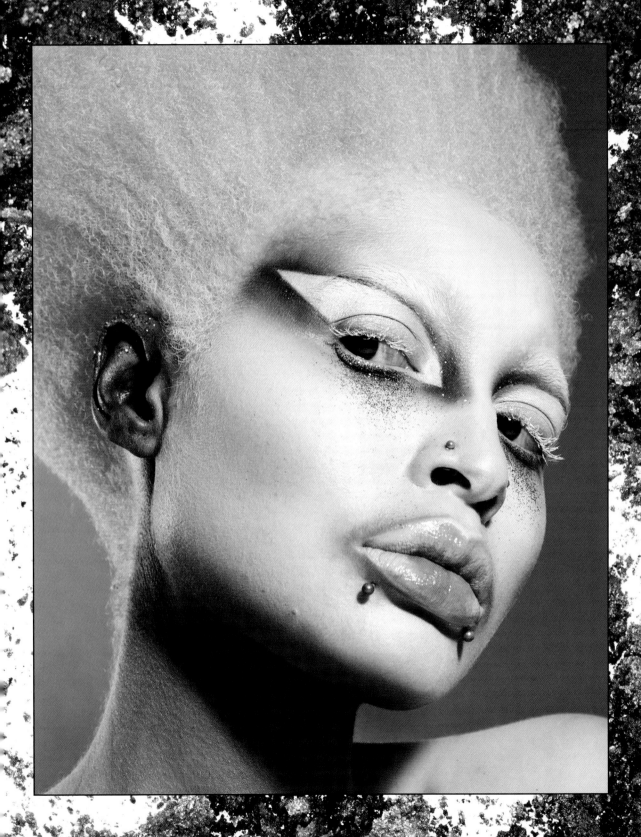

Here's how to create an editorial look based around these elements.

Apply foundation to even out the complexion, using a lighter shade of base on a sponge to brighten the centre of the forehead, under eyes, cheekbones and lip.

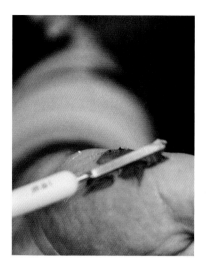

Using a large brush and soft circular motions, apply purple powder to the chin, jawline and ears.

Taking a fine eyeliner brush, add the purple liner in a geometric swoop, starting from beyond the inner corner, up around the orbital bone, out to the temples and back down to the outer corner of the eye.

Blend out the outer edge of the eyeliner with purple shadow using a small soft blending brush, working it deep into the bridge of the nose, tight under the lower lashes and up into the temple.

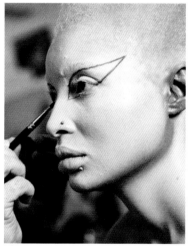

Apply purple glitter centrally under the eyes and on the tips of the ears with a flat brush. Then, using a large fluffy brush to take the purple shadow down the neck, blend into the jawline.

Filled inside the geometric eye shape with white cream and clean up any inner liner edges, then work this white through the lashes.

Line the lips using the same dark purple as the eyeliner and blend it out with a flat brush, focusing on the corners of the mouth. Mix some sheer lip gloss with the purple glitter and apply with a flat brush. Add white to this mixture and then dab on the outer edges of the lips.

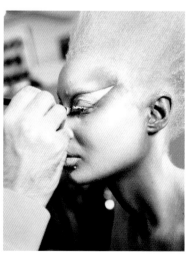

Touch some shimmery purple on the high point of the cheeks, and use a small amount of dark purple to contour under the cheekbones.

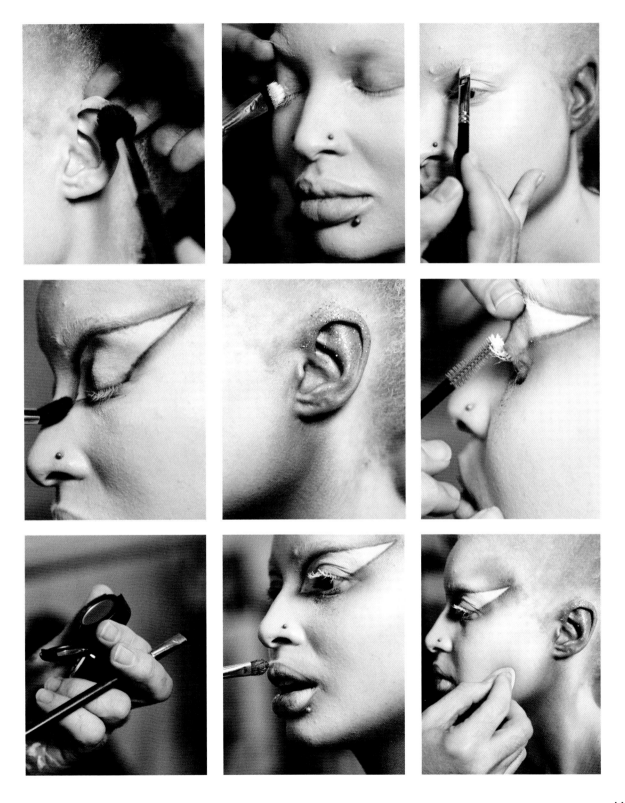

colour

The idea behind this editorial look was to use interesting and surprising colours that would not normally be seen, or which you wouldn't necessarily think could work within the same makeup. These unusual colour combinations can often be seen in the world around us, with Mother Nature effortlessly getting away with some really quite gaudy palettes; but in the material world, we tend to steer away from these clashes as they don't fit the regular overly harmonised vibe that we've become familiar with. But all that is about to change. Starting from the crazy colour chaos we created during the experiment (p.24), I zoomed in on areas that I found exciting and invigorating, colour combos which I could elaborate on and intensify to create an editorial look. While looking at these colours I was reminded of photographs from the early punk movement, the bold experimentation of avant-garde artists like Siouxsie Sioux, and I hope a little of this attitude comes across in the look.

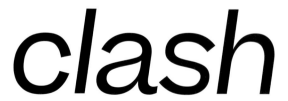

clash

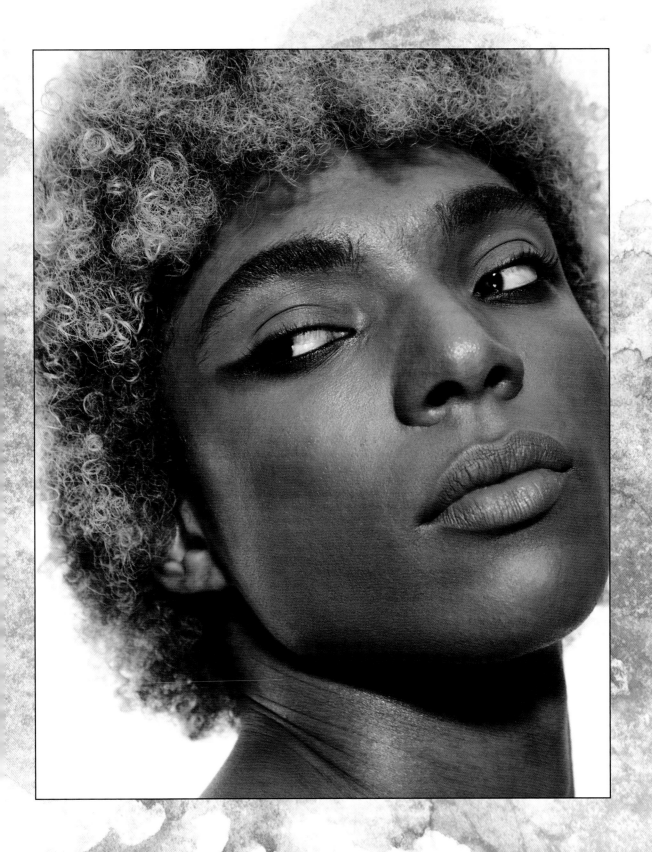

Here's how to create an editorial look based around these elements.

Using a dark brown pencil, draw around the eyes close to the lash line, extending out slightly to create a flick.

After first priming the eyelid, apply purple eyeshadow with a small dense brush onto the outer third of the eye. Swapping to a soft fluffy brush, blend the purple in towards the centre and then up towards the brow.

Apply the second colour, ochre, to the inner corner of the eye, blending towards the centre of the lid to meet the purple shadow.

Define the lower lash line with a darker shadow, blending it out to soften the edges.

Clean up any fallout from the eyeshadow and apply foundation to the skin.

With cream contour and a dense brush, use short, light strokes to deepen areas such as on and under the cheekbones.

Line the lips with a lip pencil deeper than the natural colour, then press some paler colour into the centre of the lip with a finger. Use a brush to blend the two colours together.

Finish the look with some gel brushed up and out through the brows, and a dusting of loose face powder to set the makeup.

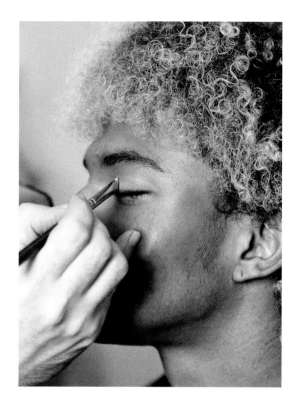

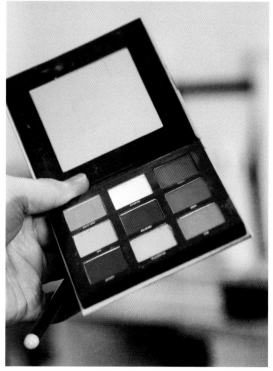

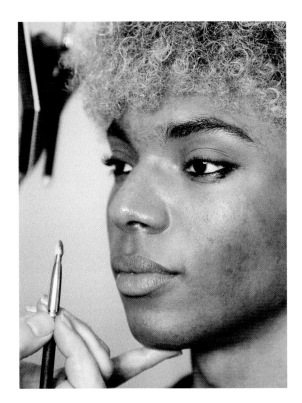

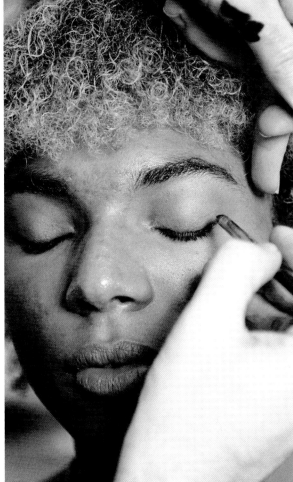

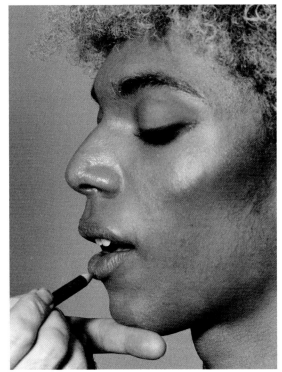

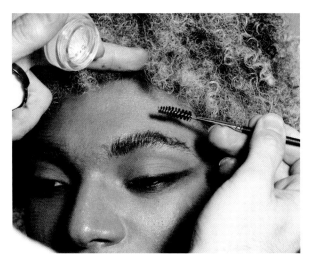

colour

For this look I needed to carefully examine the images taken during the experiment (p.28). When I was originally applying the makeup I was just looking at the tones; the lightness and darkness of the products were all I was interested in – indeed they were all I could see! However, translating this into a more considered editorial look was a real challenge. There were areas that I felt worked really well, like the blue eyeliner and the use of yellow, which is never a natural choice for me when it comes to makeup. I saw the beauty in the original application and started to dissect it. I began looking at how these light and dark tones had been applied, instead of focusing on the colours. Playing with the lip and creating this 3D ombre effect with colours that wouldn't normally go together made me excited to try other combinations in the future. I also loved the idea of creating a look that could work in both colour and through a coloured filter, or even in black and white. This experiment is a great way to gain a deeper understanding of colour values and relationships.

greyscale

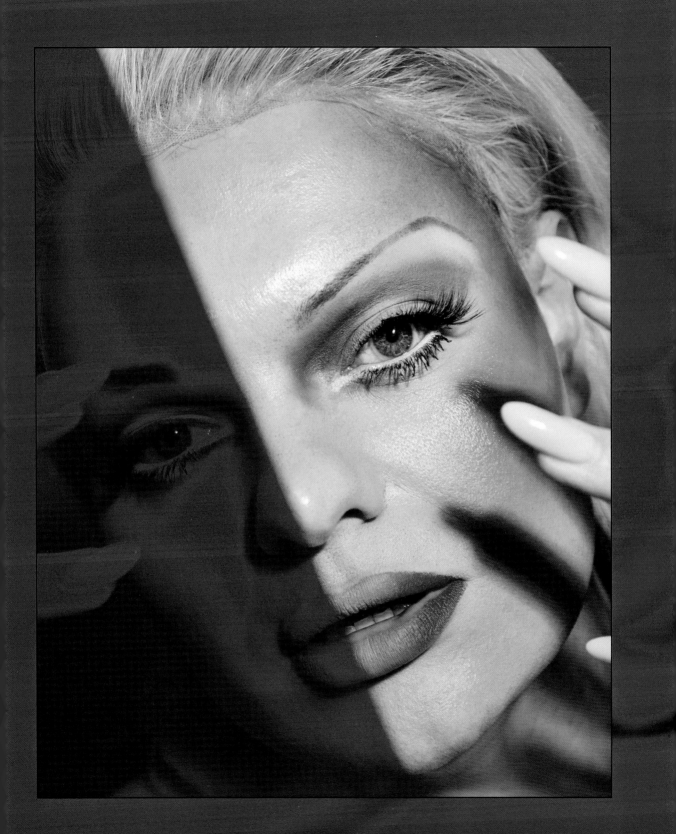

I loved the idea of creating this dramatic look.

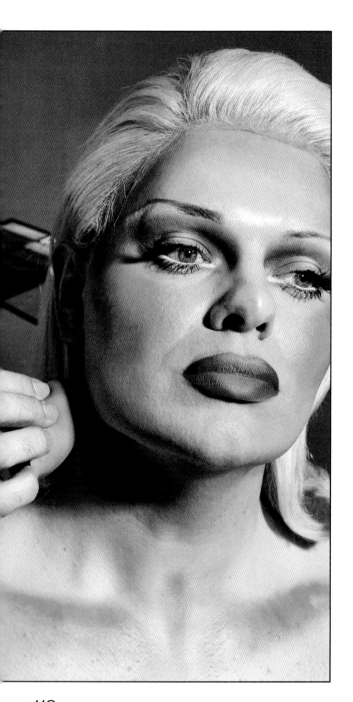

Here's how to create an editorial look based around these elements.

Apply primer to the eyelids.

Referencing the images from the experiment, create a natural contoured eye using the light and medium colours under the brow, through the socket and around the eye.

Use the dark colour at the very outer edge of the eye to create a cat-eye shape.

Using a small, angled brush, apply the darkest colour as eyeliner to the top and bottom lash line.

Add white eyeliner in the waterline and apply mascara and false lashes.

Create a contoured base by using the lightest shade on the high points of the face, deep shades in the contoured areas and medium foundation shades in between, blending them where they meet. Apply light-coloured powder to the undereye and cheeks.

To create a 3D lip, use three different lip colours with lighter shades in the centre and deeper shades around the edge, adding white powder to the centre of the lips.

Finally, draw the brows in an up-and-out direction using dark shades.

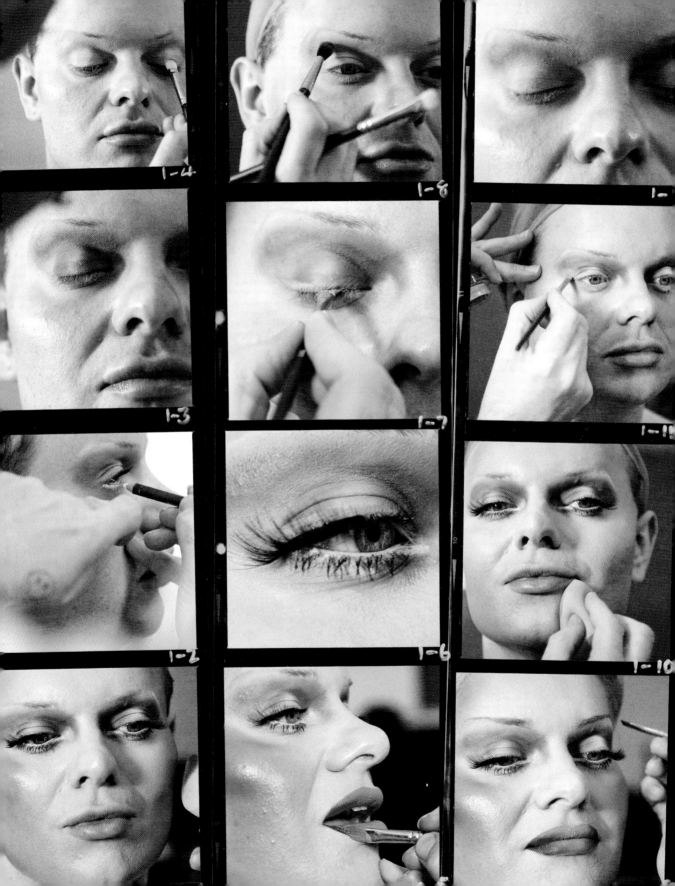

make

op

This look, like the experiment that inspired it (p.32), was so random, and entirely left to fate. What would land on the plate? Nobody knew, and that's the point. But this needn't be so limiting: if you stop looking at makeup as being for a specific use, such as lipstick, eye makeup, and so on, and begin looking at everything together as products with a particular formula – cream, powder, or liquid – then your choice becomes a lot wider. For this look I found myself with a pink lipstick, but I instantly knew I wanted to use that as a cream blush. I also got a mascara, which I knew could double up as eyeliner. How many times have you accidentally printed mascara on your lid and thought you'd ruined everything? Well, next time just add more and make it part of the look. You can really mix things up, using eyeshadows with lip gloss and adding blush with eye pencil. Though I had no idea what I would be able to use at the outset, the end result is fun, and it helps to start breaking down the makeup we have and realise what other uses we can put it to.

makeup

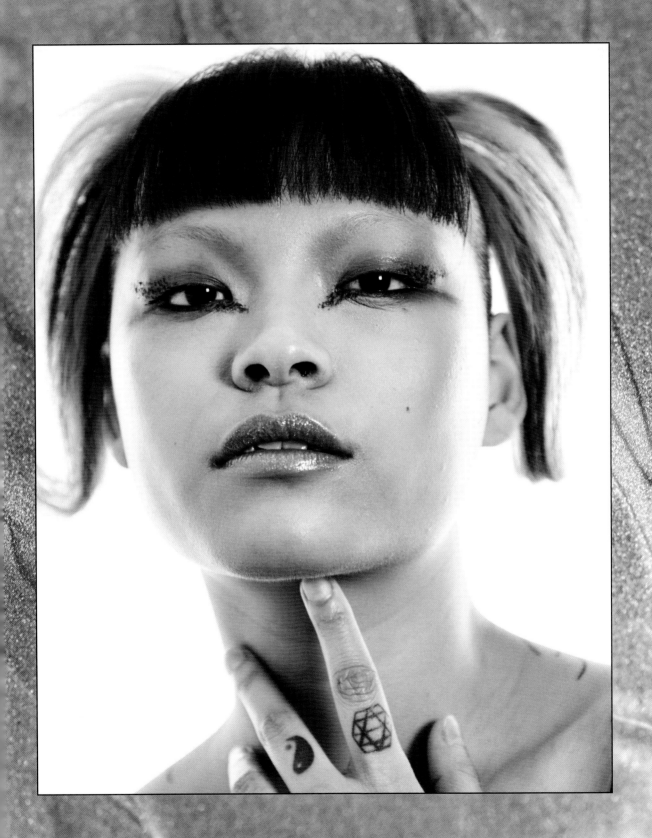

Here's how to create an editorial look based around these elements.

Apply foundation and concealer where needed to create an even base.

Take a creamy pink lipstick and apply to the outer edge of the eye, blending up towards the temple and down over the cheek.

Tap some of the mascara onto the back of the hand and use a small soft brush to apply the black liquid along the top and bottom lash line to create a smoky effect, blending out and into the pink cream.

Use the tip of the mascara wand to stipple black onto the smoked-out lines in the inner corner of the eye and at the outer edge of the upper lash line. This gives a more interesting and textured look to the eyeliner.

Lightly add the orange colour to the inner corners of the eyebrows and blend downwards slightly.

To complete the look, line the lips and apply the creamy eye colour to them before dabbing on shimmery lip oil with a finger.

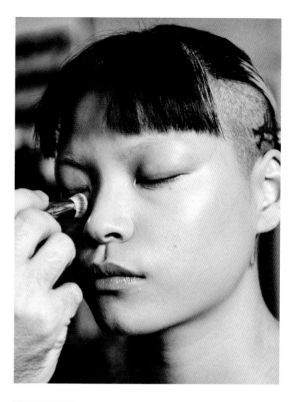

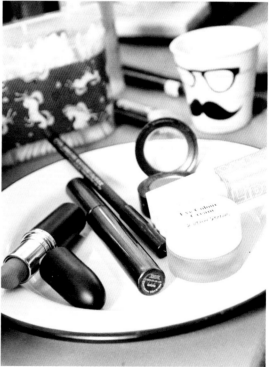

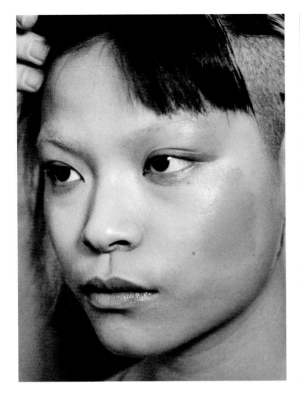

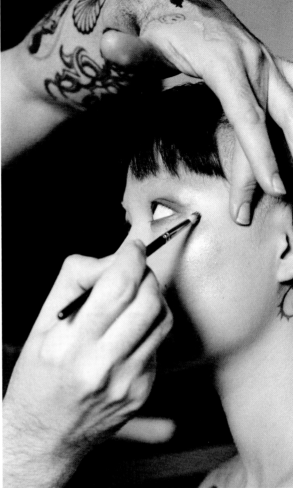

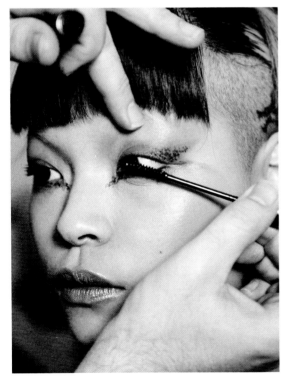

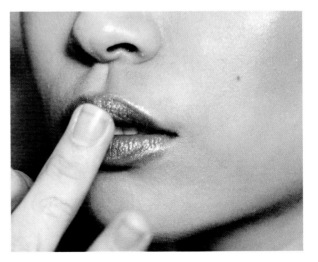

bingo

This experiment (p.36) has to have been one of my favourites to do, but it was also one of the most difficult. Surrendering the element of choice to fate was challenging enough, but passing the control of picking random products over to someone else was really hard. Maybe I thought that if I were picking the numbers, I would have some sort of cosmic power to influence the end result. I didn't, and neither did Juno, our model. We began with bingo balls, then raffle tickets, followed by the cars. To Juno's horror, no blues – her favourite colour (and my least) – had been chosen. However, this forced us both to figure how we could incorporate the selected products into a look we would love. It turned out that the colours fate had dealt us were, in fact, perfect. We should have had more faith. This look was so much fun to do, but I think we had even more fun playing the games to pick the products. Honestly, consider doing this next time you reach for your overused lippie. Leave it to chance. You might discover something new, and have a giggle along the way.

beauty

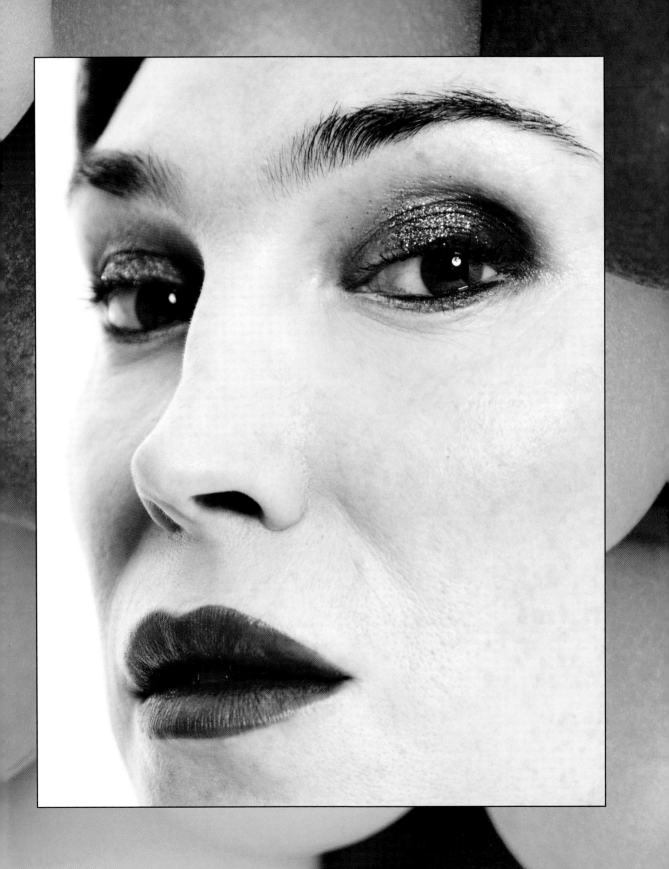

Here's how to create an editorial look based around these elements.

Using a dense brush, press the selected purple shadow onto the lid, leaving the inner third blank, then blend the colour up and out with a fluffy brush.

Apply the second shadow, a bright green, to the innermost corner of the eye.

On the inner portion of the bottom lash line, sweep a little of the bright green water-activated eyeliner.

Fill the lip with the randomly chosen lipstick – co-incidentally in this case a purple that chimed nicely with the eye colour.

Dab pink glitter onto the centre of the eye using fingertips. Clean up any fallout with tape.

Add a gentle contour to the cheeks before finishing with some setting powder where needed and lightly groom the brows.

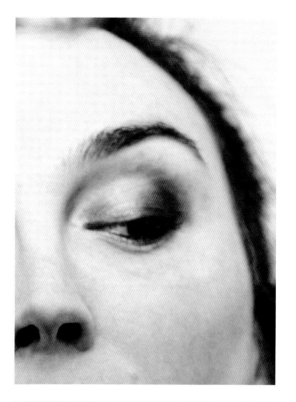

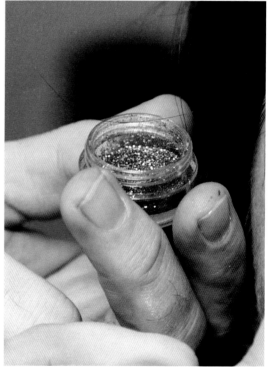

126

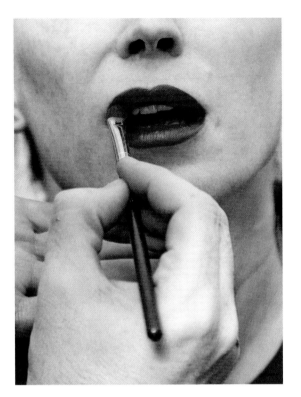
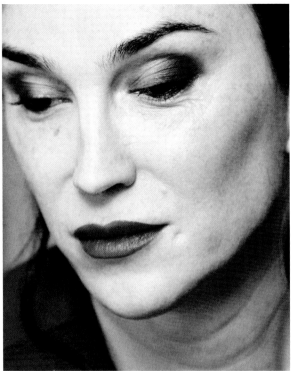
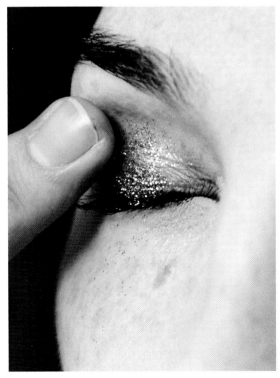
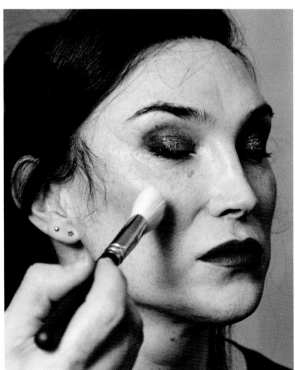

apply

When working backstage during fashion week, there's sometimes a quality to the makeup that's unlike at any other time. I've wondered if it's to do with the pressure and chaos, or whether it's the speed of application and not having time to overthink it. However, new makeup artists often struggle in this environment because they strive to get things too perfect, so the makeup can look clinical and without soul. Many times I've asked MUA's to f**k it up a little, give it a little life. This is where the idea of actually removing makeup to create a look comes into play. During the experiment (p.40) I loved how the rich colours started to melt into each other, and I wanted to emulate this within the editorial look. I also liked how the scrunched-up tissue and cotton pads left markings, so I used this technique to apply some of the makeup, particularly the highlighter on the cheek. This gave a really interesting swirl effect that was only visible when the light hit the skin. The eyeshadow has no symmetry but somehow looks just right, almost like a print design. The end result is a beautifully unique look comprised of unconventional placements.

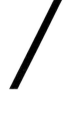

remove

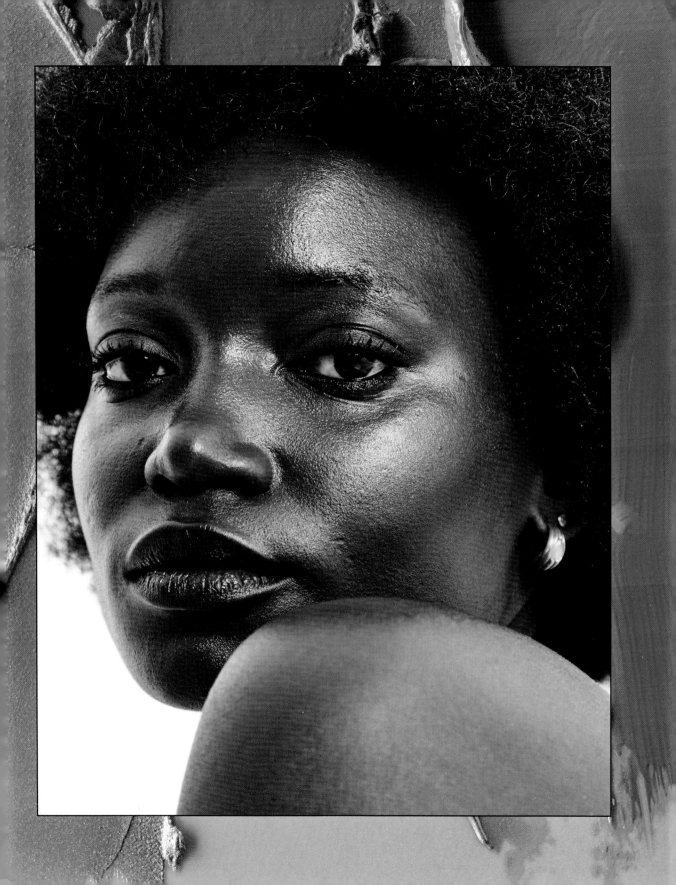

Here's how to create an editorial look based around these elements.

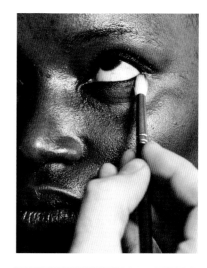

Load up the waterline and top and bottom lash lines with a black eye pencil, then use a small, firm brush to blend and soften out both lines.

Using various shades of rich, warm eyeshadow, apply the colours in no particular order to the lid and socket, avoiding symmetry, until the eye area is dressed in shadow.

Press a scrunched-up piece of tissue soaked in eye makeup remover onto the lid to gently remove some of the eyeshadow. Use a cotton swab to remove smaller areas of eyeshadow completely.

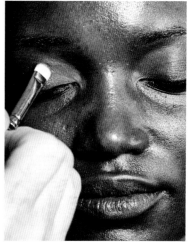

Apply mascara to the top lashes.

Using a foundation brush, add foundation to the face wherever needed to create a smooth, even base, and set with powder.

Put on lipstick as normal, then place a tissue flat over the mouth and rub a lip brush over it to blot down and partially remove the lipstick so that it looks more lived-in.

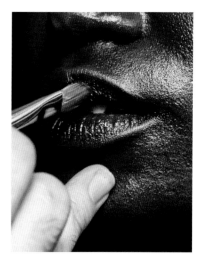

Use a cotton swab to apply small patches of black eyeshadow to the lid, and add more eyeshadow to the bottom lash line, then blend out.

Finish the look with highlighter on the brow bone and cheeks. For a more interesting effect, use a scrunched-up tissue and press into the highlighter and then onto the cheekbones.

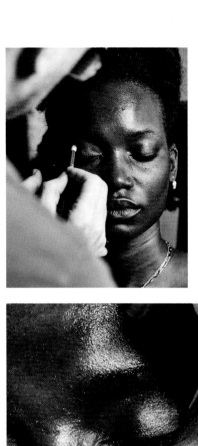
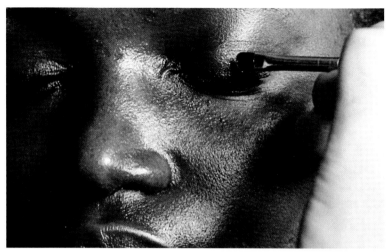
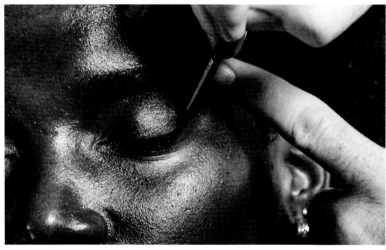
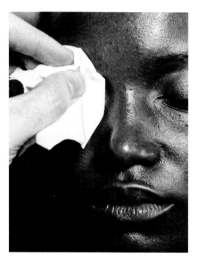
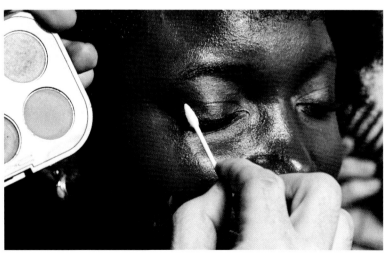
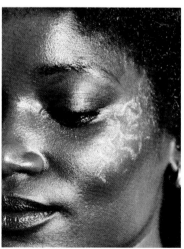

glitter

In the initial experiment (p.44), I loved the random placement of glitter in one area, where the beautiful pinks, purple and gold next to each other caught my eye. For the editorial look I had thought about mapping out asymmetrical shapes to fill with the same colours, or creating some unusual placements by laying down the cosmetic grade glitter to follow where the studio lights hit. However, I felt that in the area where I really loved the colour combinations, they looked a bit like a snake. This concept works for my model because the colours really pop against their skin tone, and their style suits something with a hard edge but with a smooth flow. When working with glitter, be aware that there's a problem no one likes to mention: blackheads. Not actual blackheads, but what appear to be blackheads. Let me explain. Glitter has a small reflective surface, and when the light hits it the colour is reflected back all bright and shiny. However, when light doesn't hit the surface it'll just look like little black dots all over the face. This means that placement is key. If you are using glitter lightly and sporadically over an area, always direct it to the high points of the face where light will most likely hit. The exception to this is when you use glitter in a dense application, which is how I use it in this editorial look.

arty

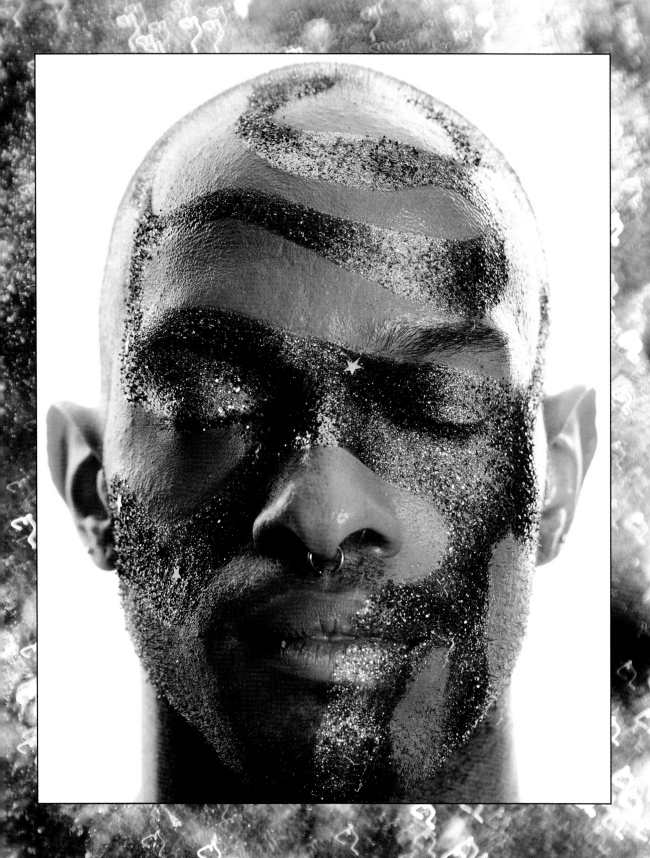

It's best to apply the foundation only after the glitter is removed...

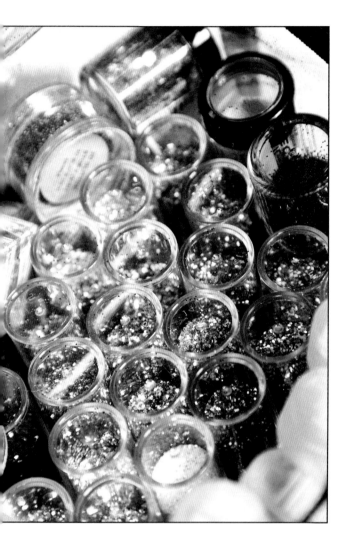

Here's how to create an editorial look based around these elements.

Using white pencil, sketch out a trail of where to place the glitter.

Apply cream within the lines where you want the glitter to adhere. The cream acts as an adhesive without the need for actual glue.

Tip out the desired shades of glitter onto a plate, then use a flat sponge to pick up and apply one colour at a time to the cream-covered areas.

Work through each of the glitter shades, slightly overlapping them to blend them together, until the area you wish to cover is complete.

Using sticky tape and a clean mascara spoolie, clean up the edges to make the design as sharp as possible.

Take a cotton bud and lash glue to apply larger pieces of glitter, like stars, and chunkier adornments such as gems.

...or it's a waste of both foundation and time.

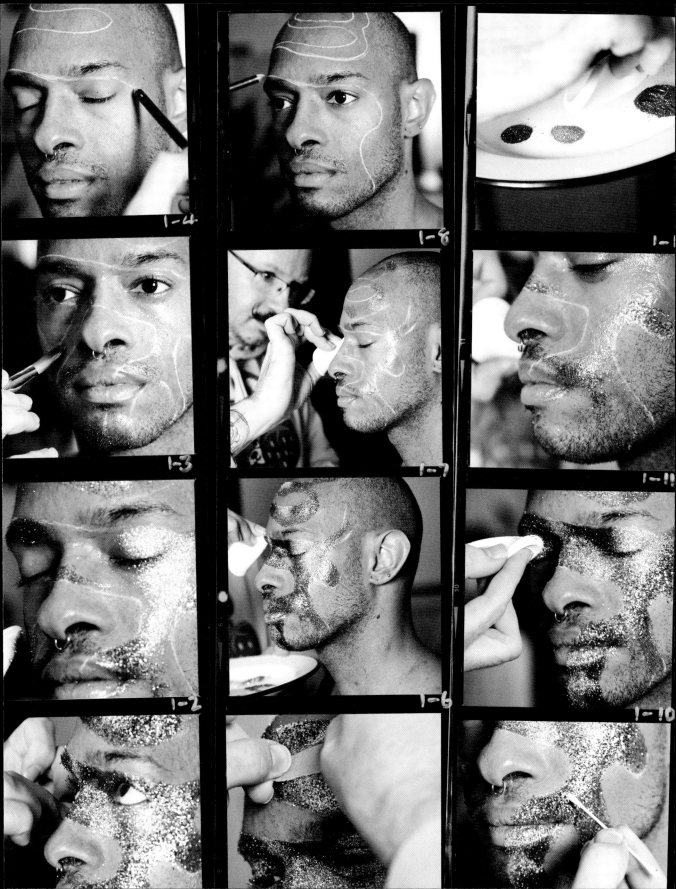

anything

but

One of my favourite things to do in makeup is to introduce elements of surprise and create moments of delight. Adding in an unexpected feature, something that makes people do a double take or even just chuckle, can elevate a mundane makeup to something that's fun, interesting and playful. You never really know what's going to work, and part of the process is figuring how you might incorporate the surprising detail into the makeup look. There were lots of trinkets that I loved playing with during the experiment (p.48), but I was most drawn to the mini pom poms. I knew I wanted to go for something bold, but I also wanted to keep it as a clean beauty look. I decided to take the conventional concept of liner and spin it to make the eyeliner out of mini pom poms. I would keep the skin minimal and give the lips a simple gloss, allowing the bold, bright colours of the pom poms to really pop and their playful texture stand out rather than being overshadowed by the rest of the makeup. Now, what inspired you most about your own experiment? And what is within arm's reach that you could incorporate into your next look?

makeup

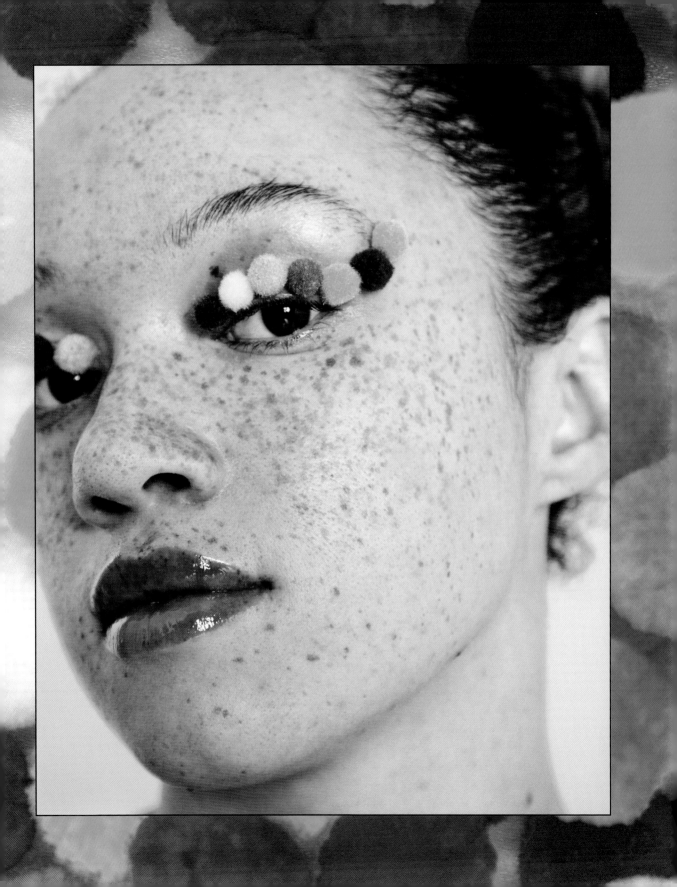

Here's how to create an editorial look based around these elements.

Begin by lightly hydrating the face and apply a little concealer as needed, then use a small fluffy brush to buff and blend the product out.

Using a pointed cotton swab, apply lash glue all along top lash line, extending out past the natural line.

Place a dot of lash glue on a very small pom pom and place at the inner corner of the lash line, using a fingertip to lightly press down and ensure it adheres.

Repeat with another differently coloured pom pom placed directly next to the first, using tweezers when it is too fiddly for fingers. Continue for the length of the glue strip, applying light pressure to secure each pom pom before moving to the next.

Allow the focus to remain on the lashes by finishing with a simple lip-plumping gloss, and use eyebrow gel to brush the brows up and out. Finally, apply a light dusting of powder to mattify desired areas.

DOM SAYS

WHEN USING ANY TYPE OF COSMETIC GLUE TO ADHERE OBJECTS TO THE SKIN, ITS ALWAYS BEST TO TAKE YOUR TIME TO REMOVE THEM. BE KIND TO YOUR SKIN AND USE SOME REMOVER ON A COTTON BUD AND SLOWLY WORK AROUND THE EDGES UNTIL THEY ARE LOOSE OR FALLING AWAY. THIS GOES FOR FALSE EYELASHES TOO.

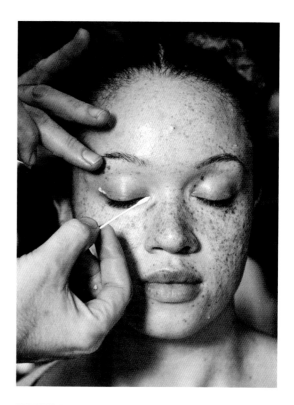

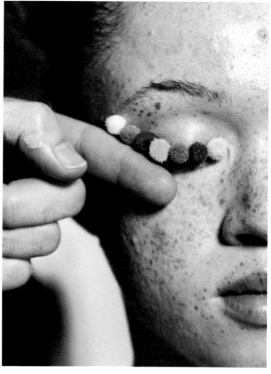

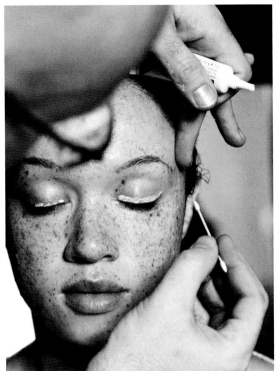

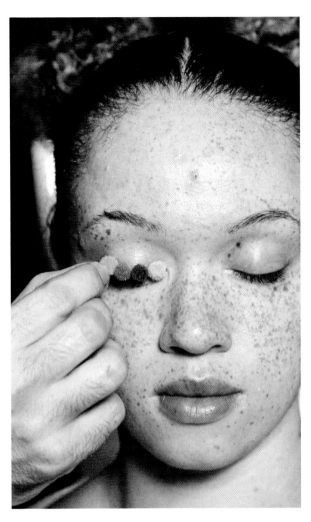

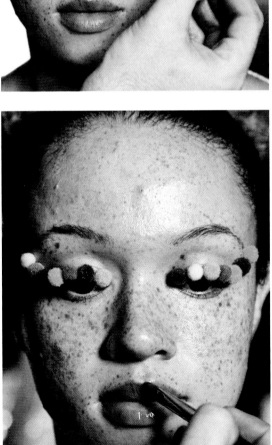

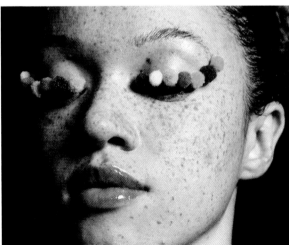

what

When doing the experiment that inspired this look (p.52), I really loved the shapes that the stars created. There was something simple and clean about them, and I knew I could use this in an interesting way. This encouraged me to go back to the stickers and look at how I could use different placements in the editorial look. I also liked the colour cluster we had produced for the relief technique. I didn't have a set plan when creating this look. It was almost an extension of the experiment, picking an element or two and taking that further to see where it went. This felt like a physical version of a spider diagram, seeing what might come out if I were to go again and again. And that is the point of makeup and art in general: never thinking that something is completely done but seeing what else you could do next time. It's a continuous journey.

a

relief!

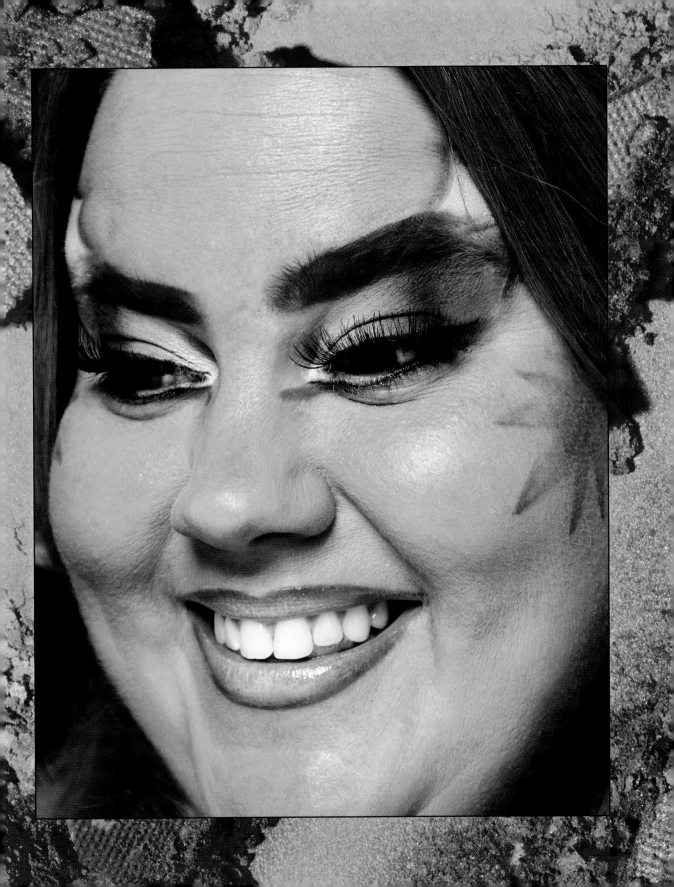

When cleaning up the edges of any patten, don't use makeup remover...

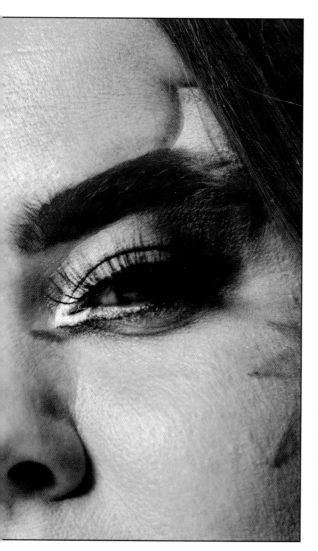

Here's how to create an editorial look based around these elements.

Prime the face and eyes to create a smooth base, then line the bottom lash line with a black pencil and smudge it out using a small brush. Apply white pencil to the waterline, and white shadow to the inner corner of the eye.

Adhere semi-circular stickers to the temples, over the inner and outer edges of the brow and up across the forehead in a continuous diagonal line. Make them as symmetrical as possible for both eyes.

Using a fluffy brush, apply white to the inner corners of the eye followed by an array of bright colours over the eyelids and up to the temple between the stickers. Remove the stickers and clean up the edges with cotton swabs.

Fill the brow with bright eyeshadows, having first placed a thin strip of cardboard just above the brow to catch any excess. Load some black onto a small, angled brush and use it to line the top and bottom lash line.

After applying foundation to the skin, add a deep blush to the cheeks. Press a shaped object onto each cheek and go over it with the foundation brush to create a silhouette, giving the blush a distinctive outline.

Give definition to the sticker outlines with black pencil, and diffuse it out with a small brush. For extra drama, curl lashes and apply mascara and a set of false lashes.

To finish, line the lips in bright pink and fill with creamy white product.

...use a little liquid foundation on a cotton swab instead.

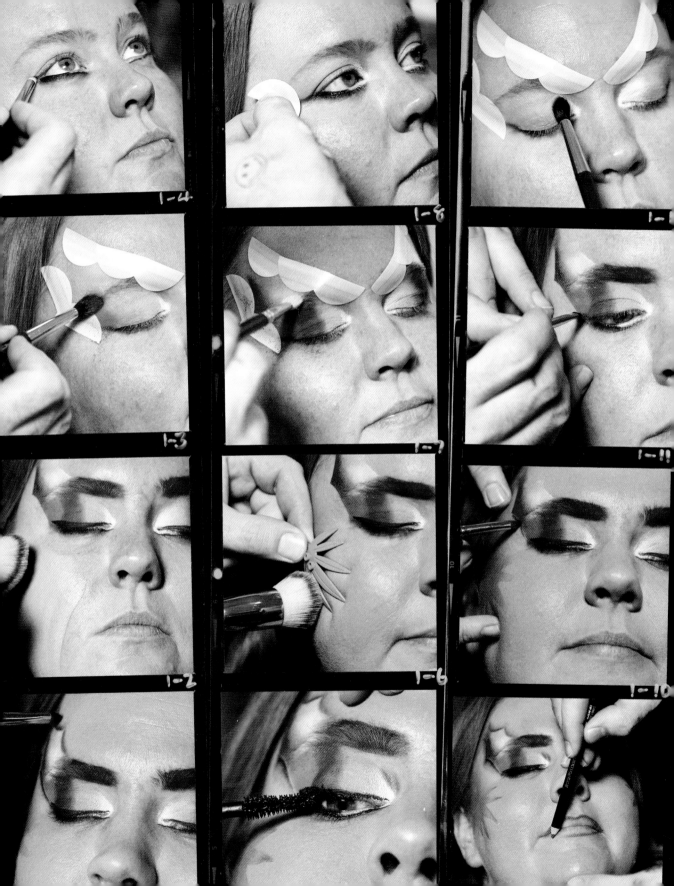

tatt -

One thing I love to do with makeup is to tease the viewer – give too much when something subtle is expected or hold back when you could easily go in full force. With this look, I wanted to show a softer side to tattoos. The old skool idea of tattoos is one of being hard, aggressive and intense. The same could be said for the tattooist and the wearer! However, tattoos have evolved and today they can be super fine, with the most delicate of lines. With this idea in mind, I went with a very simple and classic liner and lip look on a clean, fresh base, but tattoo-style. I pulled in a favour from tattooist Alex Lloyd @debutstudios and asked him to print out some amazing fine line tattoo designs, a style of tattoo using a single needle that look super fine and ultra delicate and which Alex is famed for. From this flash sheet, I used part of a barbed wire design as liner, with a couple of smaller random illustrations in the inner and outer corner of the eyes to represent smoke. Then I chose a rocket and a ruby to apply to the lip as they fitted the lip shape perfectly and would not be what people would expect. Finishing off with a thin layer of lip gloss to maintain the beauty, the Tatt-Doodle look was complete.

doodle

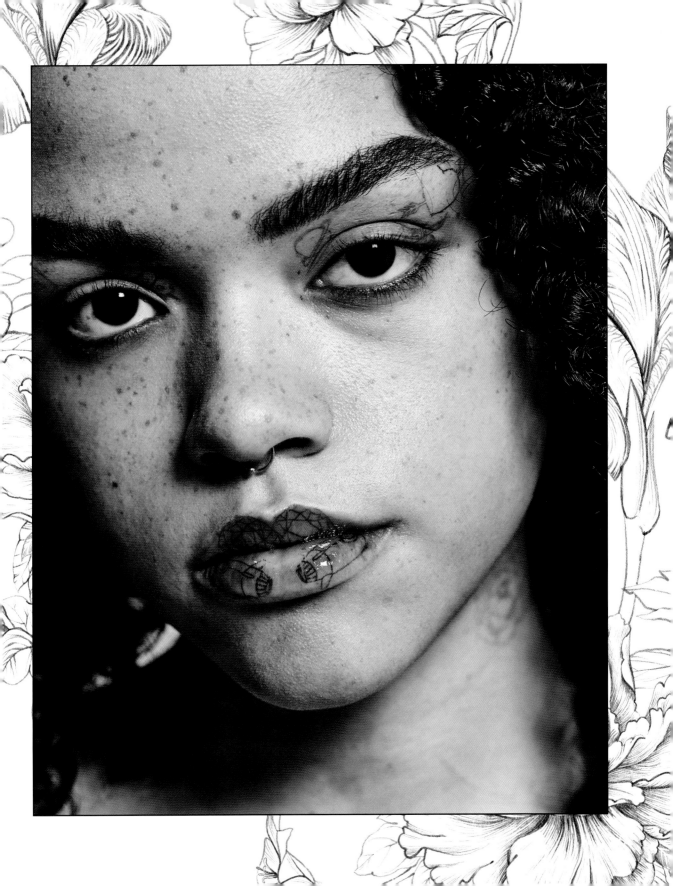

Here's how to create an editorial look based around these elements.

Remove any residual oil from the skin with a spray of alcohol on a cotton pad so that the transfers adhere better.

Following the manufacturer's application guidelines, apply the faux tattoos.

Using tweezers with a pointed end, lay the tattoos precisely over the destined area, beginning with a barbed wire design placed at the outer corners of the lids. It helps to follow the natural shapes and curves of the face with your placement, and the wire fits neatly into the contours of the eye.

Continue to work on the eyes, adding some unexpected symbols and graphics. Then carefully apply the selected rocket and ruby designs, fitting them to the natural curvature of the lip.

Apply foundation with fingertips to the naked areas of the face, and powder the entire face to mattify and set the tattoos.

Fill out the brows with powder to give the eyes a bold frame, and apply clear brow gel brushed up and out.

Apply dark eyeliner pencil to the bottom waterline and lash line only, and finish the lips with a clear gloss.

DOM SAYS

WHEN WORKING WITH TRANSFERS, INTENSIFY THE TATTOO LINES IF NECESSARY WITH AN EYELINER PENCIL OR COLOUR-IN ANY BLACK.

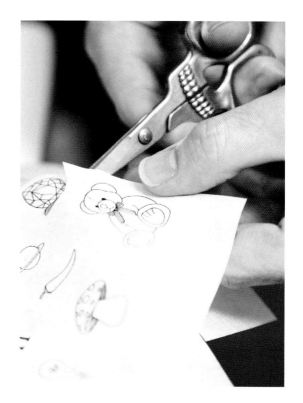

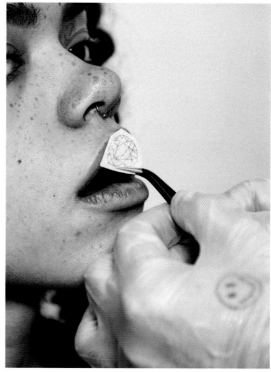

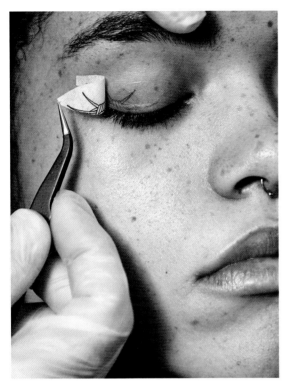

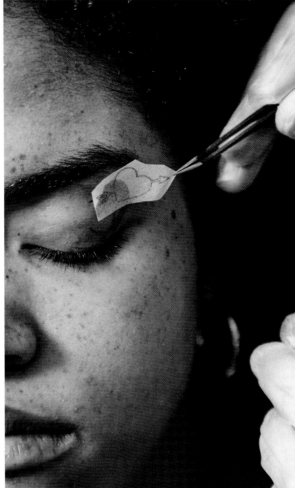

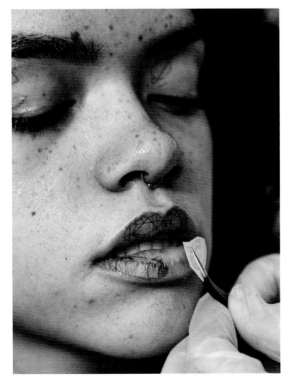

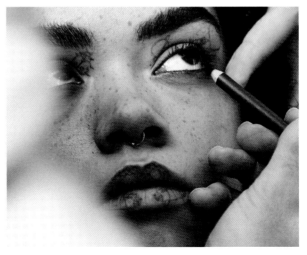

get your

I'm not going to lie; this look was tricky. The desire to pick up a makeup brush to finesse and refine the look throughout the application was strong! A lot of willpower was required in order to not grab a tool. However, I stand by my original comment (p. 60) that fingers and hands can be your best friends when applying makeup, allowing you to achieve a well-blended look that has a human touch. The focus of this look was actually the formula of the products rather than the colours or finish. When carrying out the experiment you will have no doubt discovered that, when using only your hands, creamy products are often easiest to work with. So the makeup needed to have a cream base – at least to begin with, as some cream-based products do dry down to a rigid waterproof finish. As we could use only fingers, powders were not going to blend out as easily as they would using a brush. Fingers can smoosh creams out and blend them into each other. One thing you do lose is precision: it's not easy to get symmetry and there is a lack of refinement. However, you do gain a tactile quality and a control that you don't get with brushes. You get to feel the face and almost instinctively know where things should go.

hands

dirty

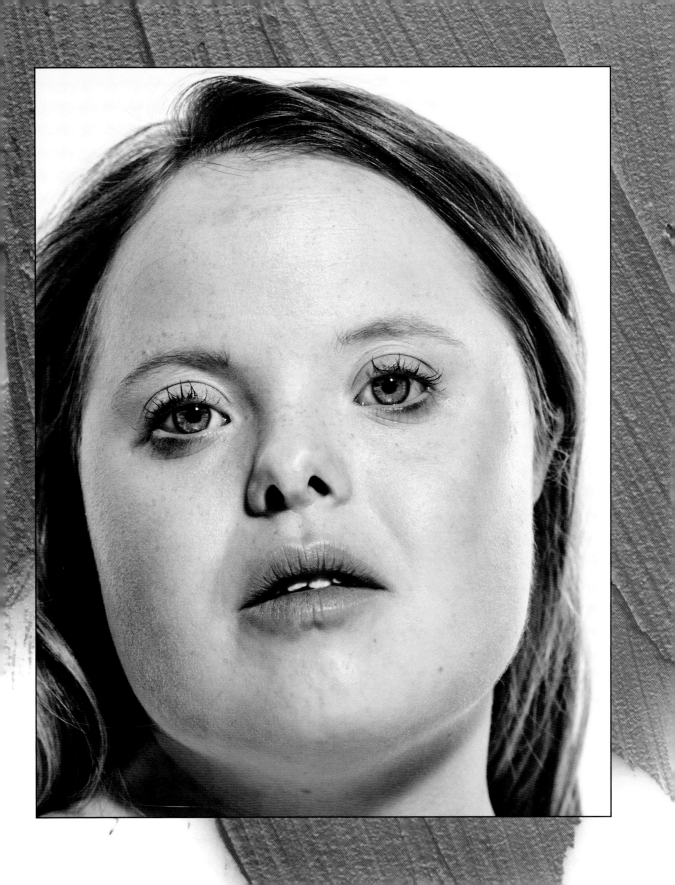

Here's how to create an editorial look based around these elements.

Using only fingers, gently apply concealer under eyes, at the centre of chin and around the nose, lightly patting the product in.

Create a flushed cheek by applying lipstick to the heel of the hand (inside of the hand between thumb and wrist), then rubbing the product between the heels of both hands. With palms facing out, place your thumbs above your ears and lightly roll the heels of the palms down the cheeks towards the mouth. Use fingers to diffuse the edges of the colour.

Gently tap pale blue shadow onto the eyelids, using a fingertip to blend it upwards. Apply the same shade underneath and blend with fingertips. Build up intensity on the outer corner of the eye by patting on more shadow.

Use a darker blue eye pencil to line the eyes along the top and bottom lash line then smudge out with a finger. When applying an eye or lip pencil, give it a little rub on the back of your hand to help warm it up for easier application.

Sweep pale pink lipstick onto the lips, and layer a brighter pink over the top in the centre of the lip.

Use an eyebrow pen to give added definition to the brow, and the look is finished.

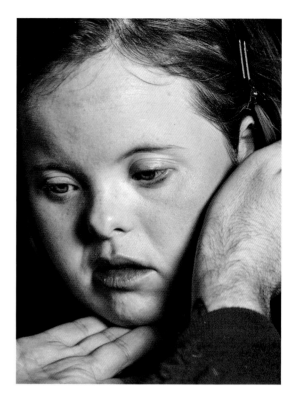

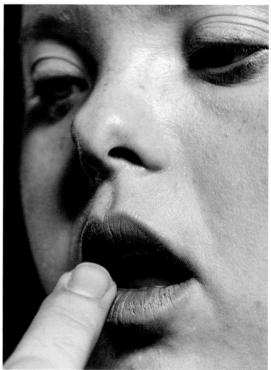

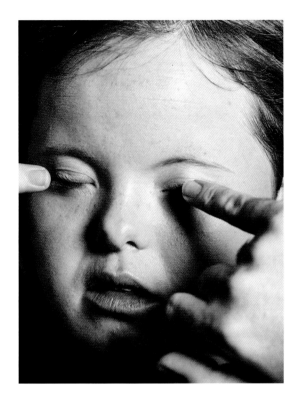

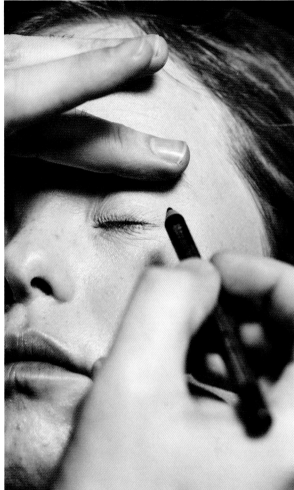

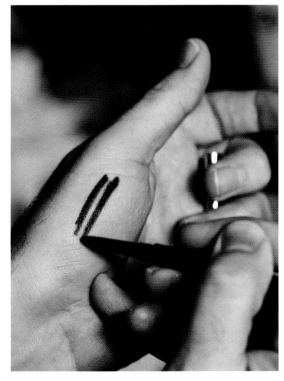

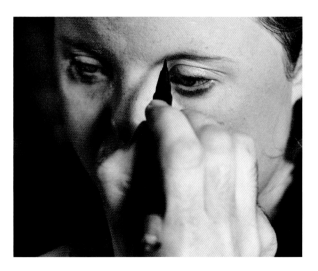

print

I do like a cheat. If there's something I can do or use that might deliver a simpler and quicker result, then I am in. While playing around during the experiment (p.64), I noticed how the empty pill packet delivered a repeat dot effect, much like in a comic book or in Lichtenstein's Pop Art images. This discovery led me to look at the process colours (cyan, magenta and yellow) I was using for the experiment in a different way. I wanted to layer these colours as they might appear in a traditional printing process, and repeat the dots around the face, creating subtle colour changes where they accidentally cross over. When creating the look I could have spent time mapping out a grid to work out where the dots should be positioned; I could have painted each one individually, looking for consistency and precise edges; I could have spent hours applying and reapplying the design to achieve perfect symmetry. OR I could just use an empty pill packet as a stamp and do the whole look in 30 minutes! Adding a layer of printed makeup to any look can be a fun way to add a design element while also being super simple to achieve.

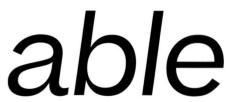

able

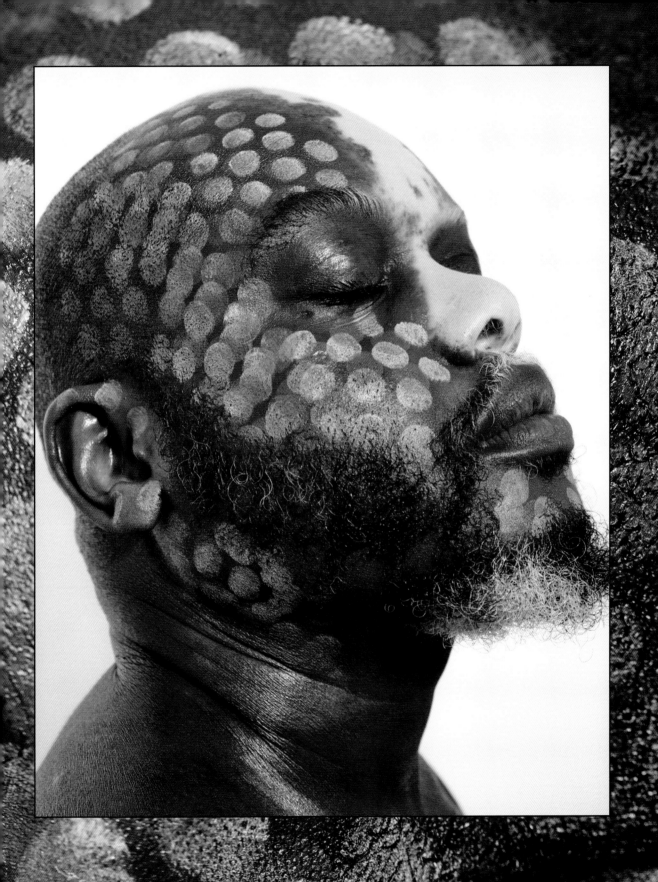

Here's how to create an editorial look based around these elements.

Hydrate the face and lips with moisturiser and lip conditioner, then apply concealer and foundation where needed.

Using a firm flat bush, apply an even coat of pink paint over a blister pack of pills and press it firmly onto the face at the side of the forehead

Continue on both sides of the face, stamping a uniform pattern of dots.

After wiping the packet clean, repeat this process using yellow, mapping the placement to slightly offset where the pink dots have already been printed.

Repeat the process using blue, again slightly offsetting the stamping so that the colours overlap a little.

Finish with eyebrow gel to brush the brows up and out, and set with a translucent powder and misting spray to prevent smudging and help the makeup to stay put for longer.

DOM SAYS

TRY VARYING THE DENSITY OF THE DOTS BY USING DIFFERENT LEVELS OF PRESSURE TO ACHIEVE DIFFERENT EFFECTS.

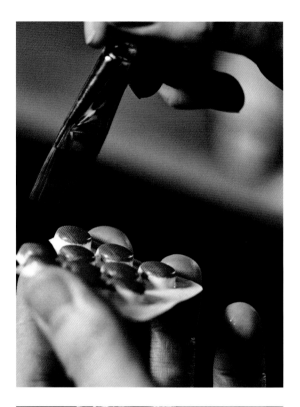

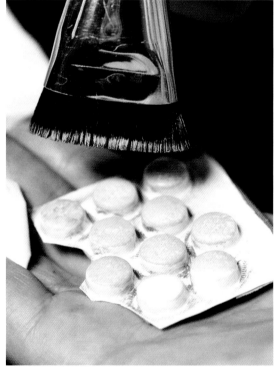

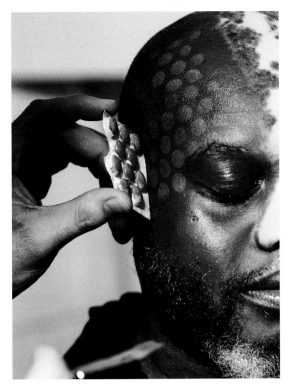

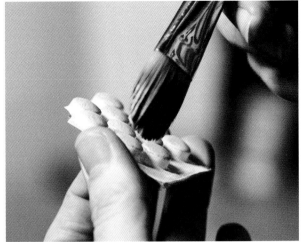

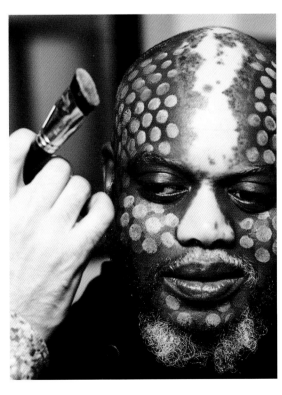

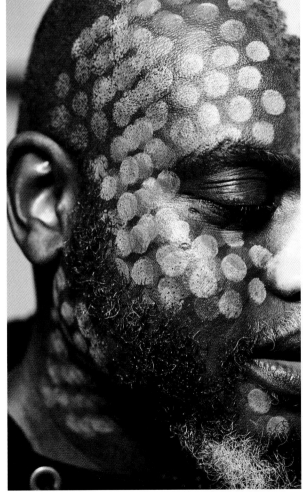

tool

What's great about the experiments in this book is that you can do them any number of times and end up with an unexpected and unconventional result on every occasion. When carrying out this experiment (p.68) you could apply makeup using any random tool from the kitchen and each time it would produce an entirely different result. There is no end to how exciting, brilliant and fun makeup can be if approached in an unusual way. For this look I wanted to focus on the eyes, and had noticed in the experiment that the spoon hugged the eye shape wonderfully. The shape meant that the spoon did 99 per cent of the work. I wanted to use colours that would give a vaguely 1960s feel – think London's Carnaby Street – so I layered yellow, green and blue. These analogous shades (next to each other on the colour wheel) work well together, allowing the viewer to focus on the model's eyes without being distracted by anything clashing on the lids. The layered shades led me to select an opposite peachy colour for the lip.

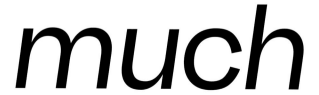

too

much

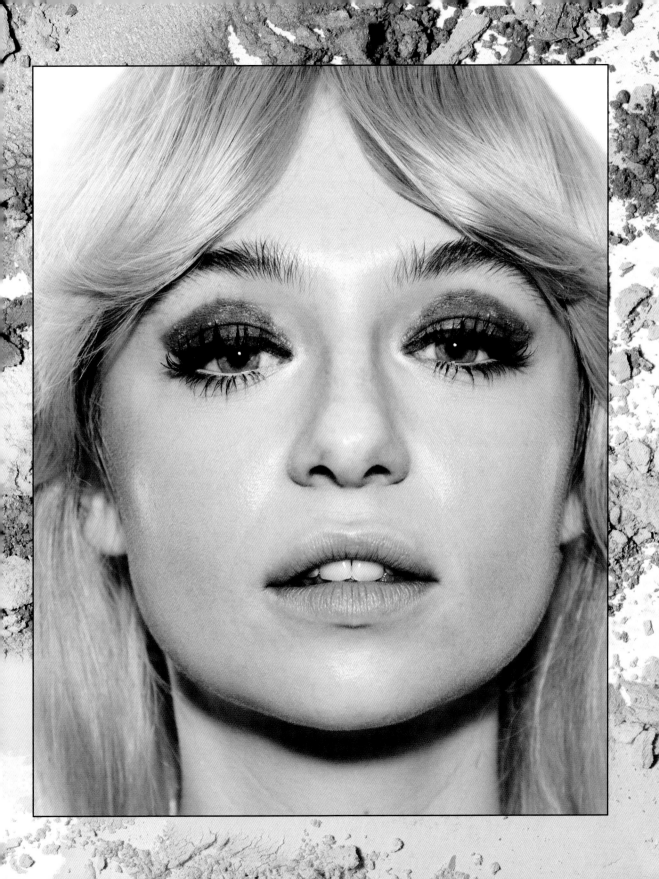

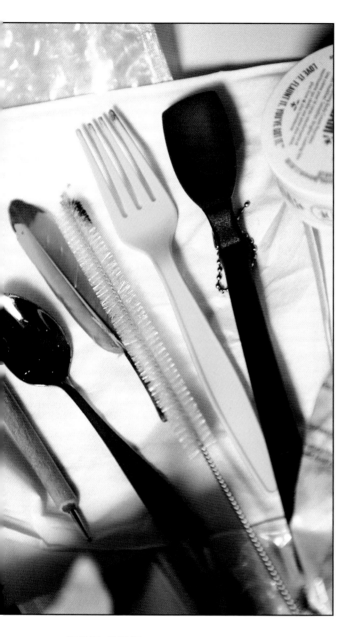

Here's how to create an editorial look based around these elements.

Begin by using the back of a spoon to spread a dark greige cream makeup paint over the eyelids and just below the bottom lash line.

Take a deep blue makeup paint and, again using the back of the spoon, press it in non-uniform patches onto the eyelids.

Repeat this pressing technique using yellow cream, allowing the pigment to create a textured effect rather than smoothing it out. Make sure to also place the yellow onto the bottom lash line, focusing the pigment in the inner half (use the tip of the spoon to achieve more accurate placement).

Use black liner and a small, angled brush draw liner onto the top lash line and extend in an outward flick.

Add white eyeliner pencil all around the waterline and to the inner corners of the eyes, and apply two coats of mascara to the top and bottom lashes.

Clean up any spills around the eyes using a cotton swab and then apply foundation to the skin with a brush.

Dab peach lipstick in the centre of the lips and rub them together to blend it out, then apply cream blush to the cheeks using the back of the spoon, gently tapping to soften the edges.

Brush brows up and out, and set with eyebrow gel. Apply face powder with a puff to set under the eyes and to mattify the T-zone.

DOM SAYS

I COULD REDO THESE EYES MULTIPLE TIMES AND THE RESULTS WOULD LOOK COMPLETELY DIFFERENT EVERY TIME. THAT'S WHAT IS SO FUN ABOUT USING UNCONVENTIONAL TOOLS.

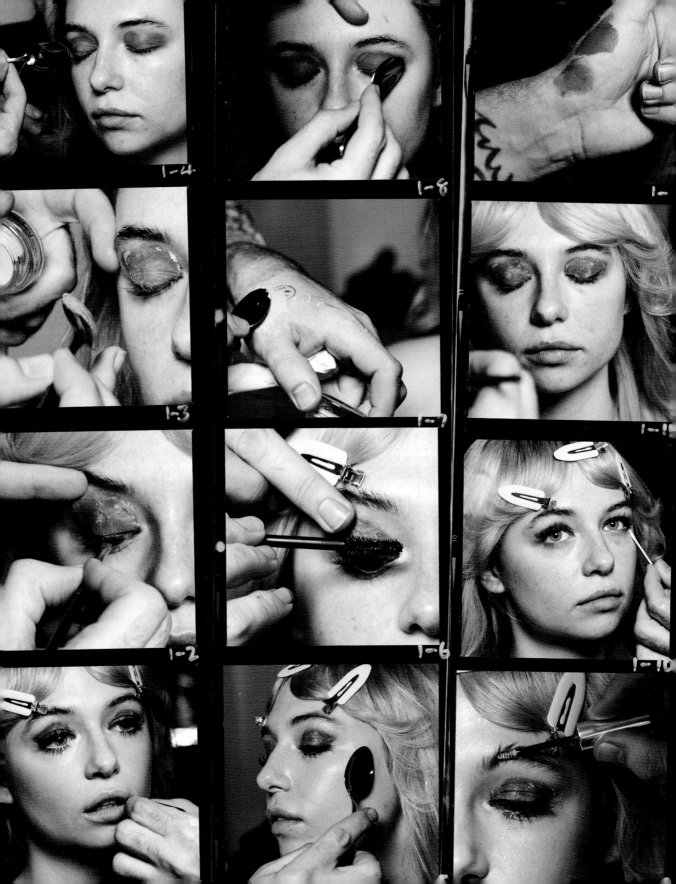

opposites

The idea of using both hands to apply makeup might seem silly to most people. Makeup, with its demand for precision and symmetry, requires a steady hand and a high level of control. However, it's precisely this control that can get in your way when trying to break free from the constraints of perfection. Now, I'm not saying that perfection isn't something that should be aimed for. It's just unfortunate that striving for perfect application can end up being our focus, and this prevents us from fully embracing creativity. What I enjoyed most about the experiment was the fluidity of the application, of not really knowing where I was going but letting the movement of the brushes guide the design. There is a beauty that comes from this organic movement, from being able to truly let ourselves go in the moment and allow our subconscious to lead us. I wanted to bring this flow to the look, but in a slightly more considered way. Using the non-dominant hand can provide the little quirks and micro-imperfections that can deliver a more interesting makeup look.

attract

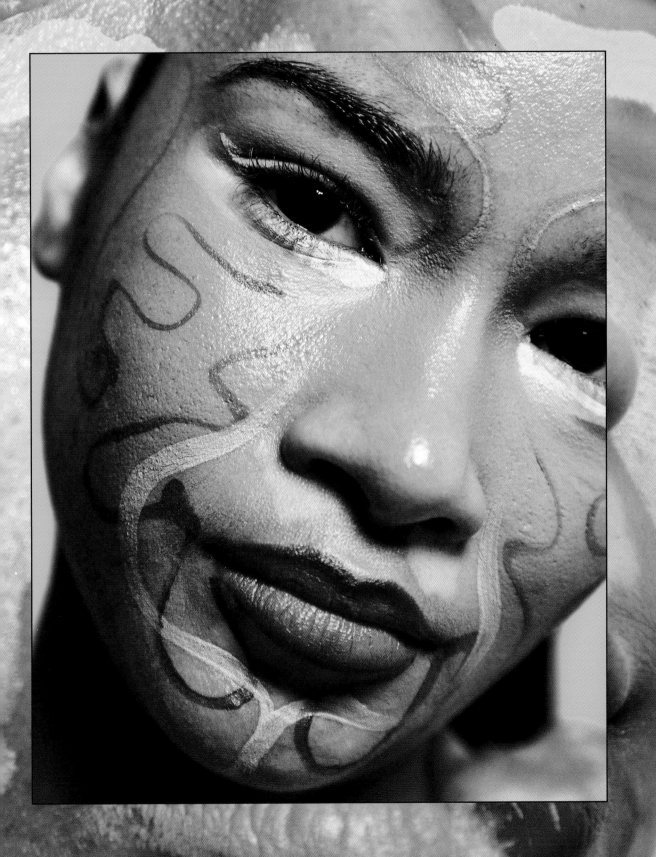

Break free from the constraints of perfection.

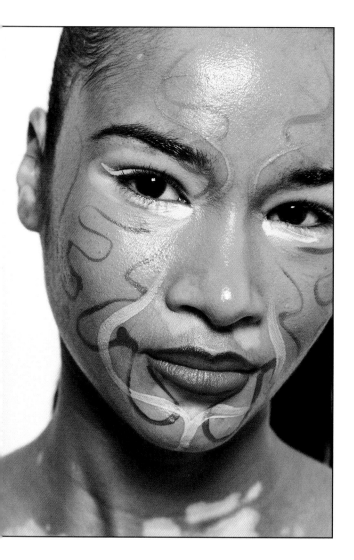

Here's how to create an editorial look based around these elements.

Apply your base in whatever style you like.

Using a fine tipped brush and picking from a colourful water-activated colour pallet, load it with one colour.

First, using your non-dominant hand, draw a flowing line in one area of your face and then replicate this line, mirrored on the other side of the face with your dominant hand.

After cleaning the fine-tipped brush, repeat the process on another section of the face with a different colour in the palette. Repeat this process, cycling through the colours of the palette but keeping the colours distinct.

Don't worry about lines overlapping; play with using lines on different sections of the face.

Finally, line the lips and fill in with a bright shade using a lip brush.

DOM SAYS

ALWAYS LEAD WITH YOUR NON-DOMINANT HAND, THEN REPLICATE USING YOUR DOMINANT HAND. THIS ALLOWS YOU MORE FREEDOM OF FORM, AS YOUR DOMINANT HAND WON'T BE CALLING THE SHOTS.

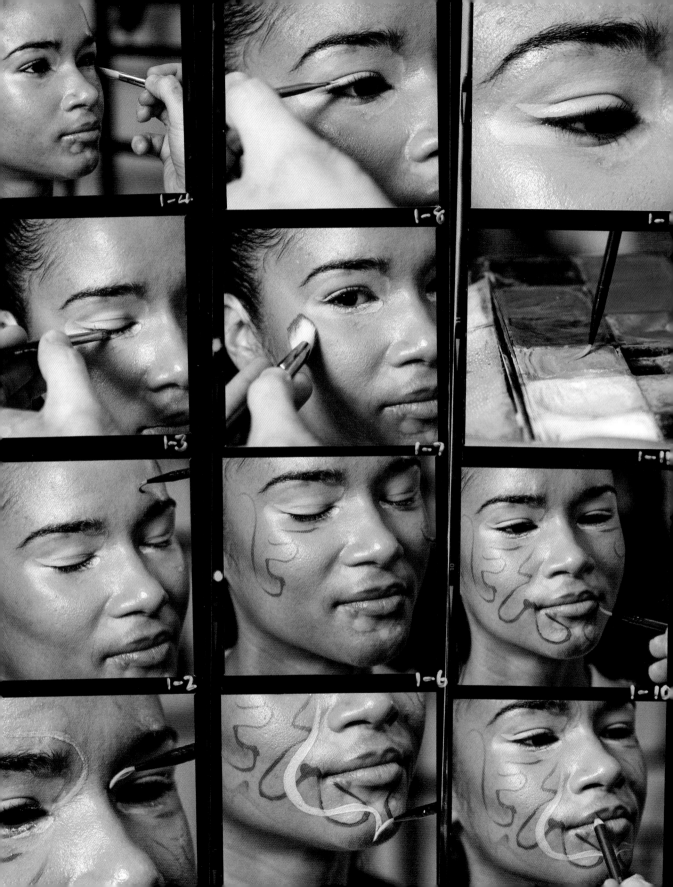

sweet

shop

When playing with the original experiment of sweet shop beauty (p.76), I just loved so many of the colours and the random overlays of tones and shades and intensities. This inspired me to give each feature on the face its own unique look. Just as a sweet shop is a clash of colours and designs, the face would also. Consider the face a recreation of its very own sweet shop. Applying different colour theory colour groupings and application techniques, I went with graphic liner, to soft muted blends and finally a contrasting pop. The idea was to create a look that was bold and eclectic while also being fun and tempting. Plus there was a lot of sugar pulsing through me while doing this look. Waste not, want not!

beauty

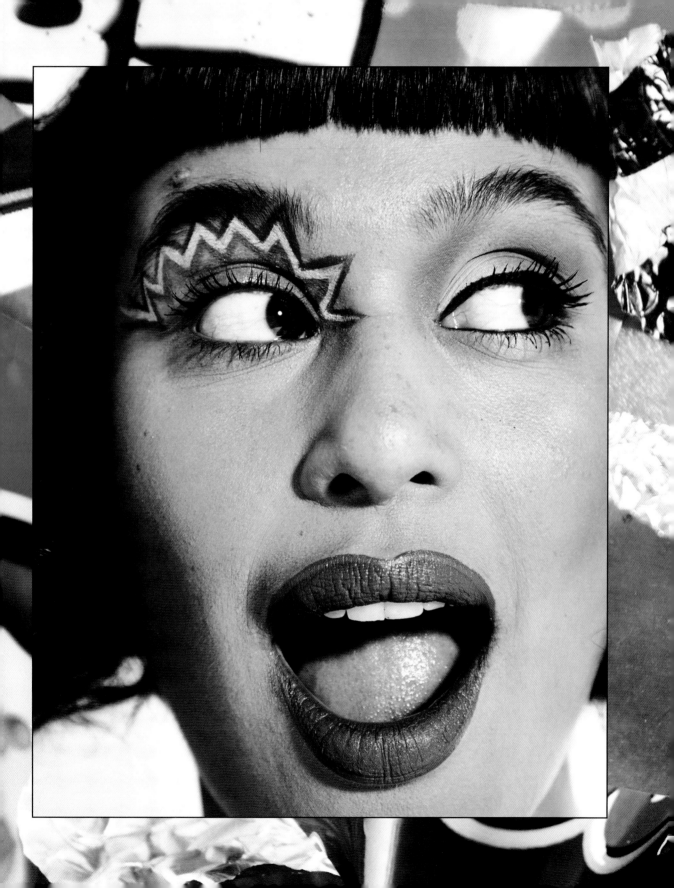

Here's how to create an editorial look based around these elements.

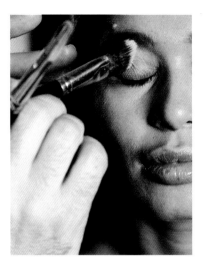

Start by using concealer and foundation to create an even base.

Apply a sugar pink blush over the apples of cheek, blending along the cheekbone and adding a little on the chin.

On the left eye, apply yellow eyeshadow to the inner half of the eyelid, and bright pink to the outer half and innermost corner, blending up and out. Use the same colours under the eye. Where the two shades meet, blend until a soft orange is created. Apply mascara to finish.

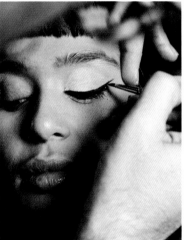

With an angled brush and black eyeliner, create a winged flick, using a black eye pencil to wrap around the waterline.

On the right eye, use a small brush to draw a zigzag line just above the right eye socket in yellow.

Before finishing the eye, mix a creamy red and blue on the back of the hand to create purple and apply this to the lips, then use bright orange with a fine brush to line them.

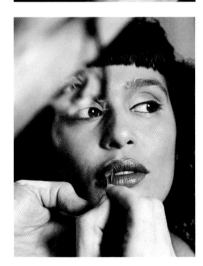

Returning to the eye, draw a blue zigzag underneath the yellow one, adding a little flick at the inner corner of the eye. Finish with a line of red above the yellow.

Brush the brows up and out with eyebrow gel, and use an eyebrow pen to draw thin lines as shadows to create a more natural brow.

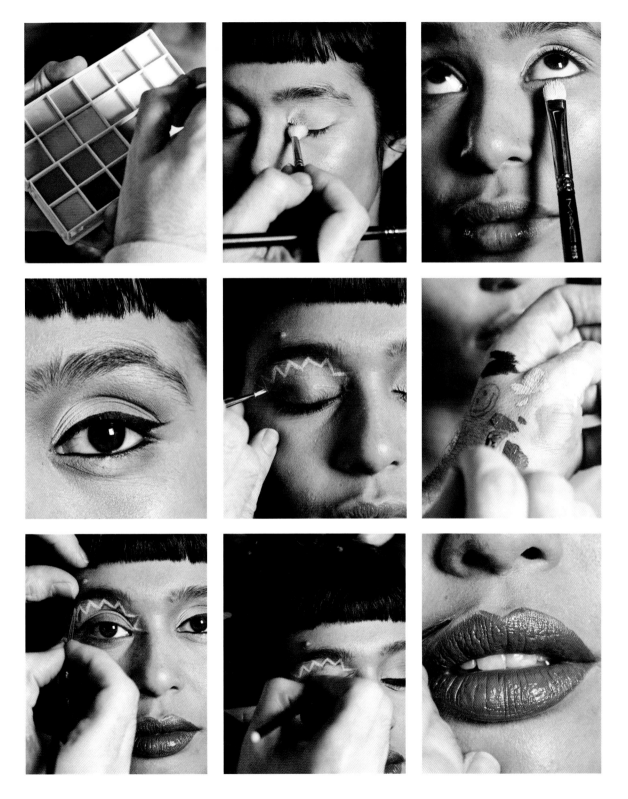

When working with clashing colours, you don't need to apply them in equal amounts. Using just a small dash of the opposite (complementary) colour will allow the eye to see them more intensely.

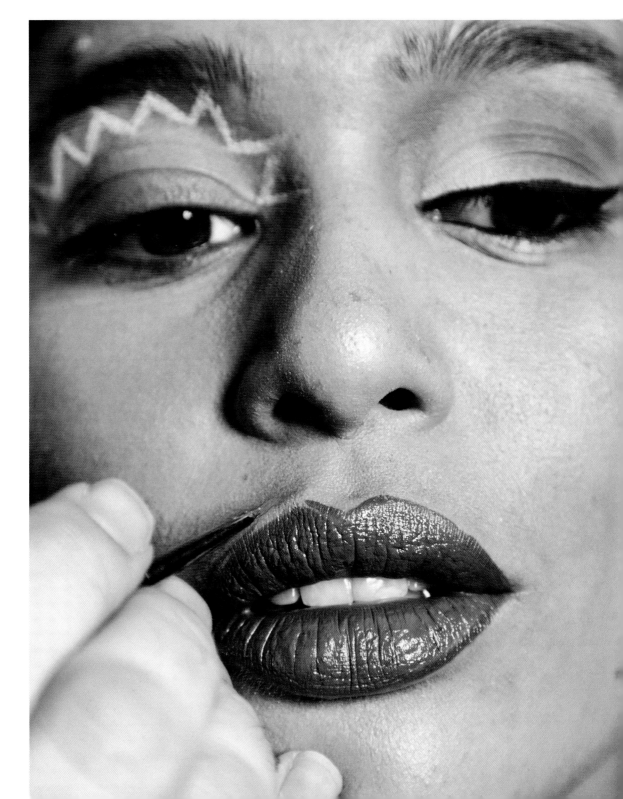

art-

Art has always played a big part in my life, and never more so than when I moved from studying fine art and sculpture to makeup. I have always been influenced by artists from other mediums, and when looking for inspiration in a wide range of art movements during the experiment for this look (p.82), I recalled that the first artist to really capture my imagination, over 30 years ago, was the Dutch painter Piet Mondrian. I loved his stripped back abstraction, clean lines, primary colours and geometric compositions. Thinking about this made me wonder how I could incorporate these ideas within the constrictions of facial features: how to create straight-looking horizontal and vertical lines around the curvature of the face; where to place colour blocking, and where to leave the natural skin tone. This was such a fun look to do, and it forced me to question my natural flow of symmetry and balance while maintaining precision. Art will continue to inspire me, which is why I spend just as much time in galleries as I do in beauty halls.

like

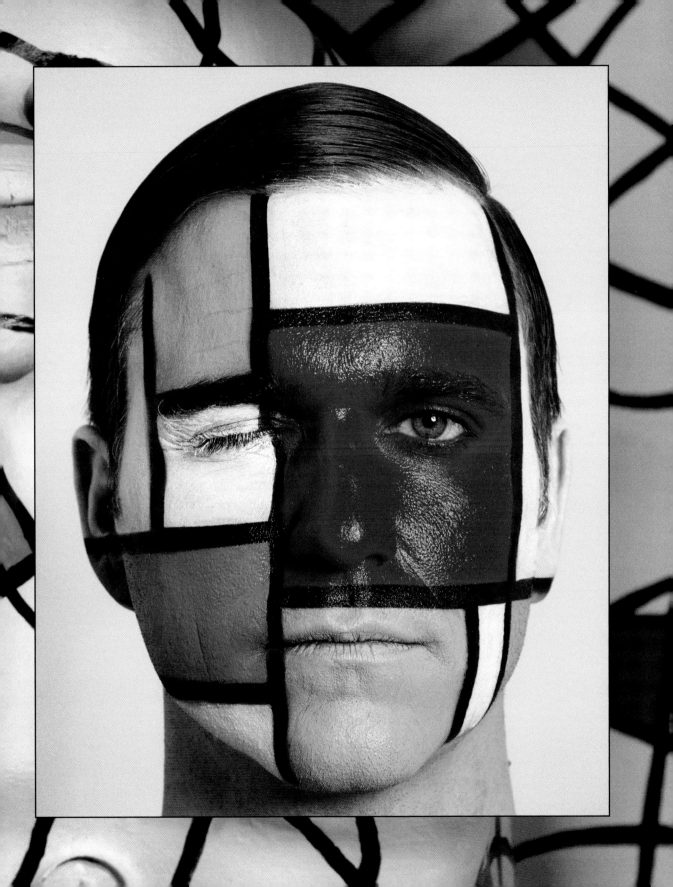

Here's how to create an editorial look based around these elements.

First, map out grid areas on the face with an eye pencil, judging by eye the placement of straight guidelines on a round face while looking directly into the mirror. A series of short pencil strokes can be easier than attempting a continuous straight line.

Use a small brush to pick up some black cream and draw over these rough outlines, making a bolder line over the top, and then use a cotton swab to clean up the edges.

Randomly fill in some of the squares with red, blue and white paint, leaving some squares blank.

Finally, in the blank squares add a little foundation and concealer to even out the skin tone in those areas.

DOM SAYS

CREATING STRAIGHT LINES FREEHAND TAKES PRACTICE AND A STEADY HAND. BEGIN LIGHTLY, KEEPING YOUR GUIDELINES FAINT, AND CONTINUALLY EVALUATE AS YOU GO, MAKING ADJUSTMENTS BY ERASING AND REDRAWING IF THE LINE FEELS LIKE IT BEGINS TO DEVIATE.

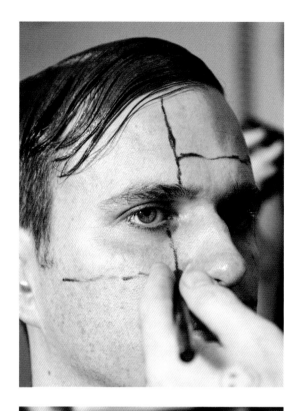
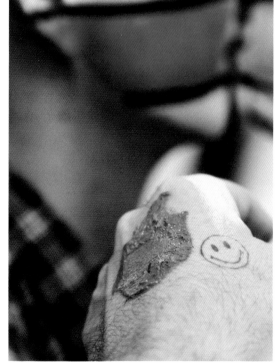

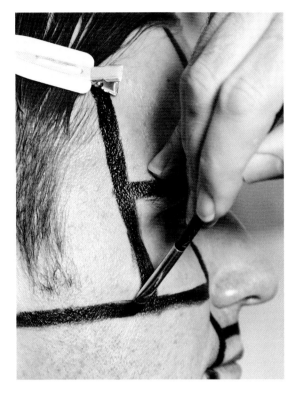

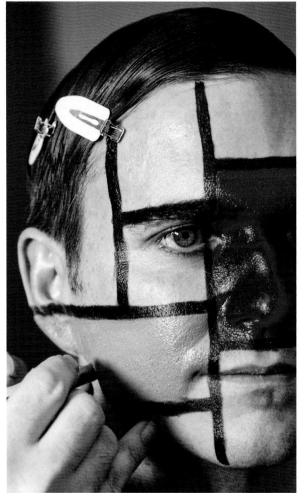

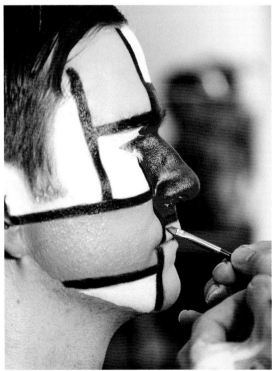

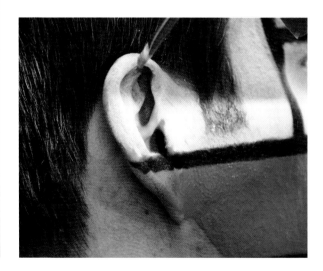

in tune

with

During the experiment that inspired this look (p.86) I was entirely guided by the music I was listening to. It was at first joyful, then rhythmic, then fresh and light. The colours were randomly chosen, and so was the placement. I let the music dictate what was happening. I wanted to take the colours I had been inspired to use around the eyes and employ them in a more flattering way in this look. Think of it as being a bit like taming a freestyle jam session into a more considered musical composition. The teal and aqua shades would not necessarily have been my first choice, but they really worked with the model's eye colour and skin tone. The lip was a bright note set against the electric blue noise of the eyeshadow. Colour can be intimidating, but the surge of joy you feel when using them in your makeup can be just as powerful as the emotional punch you get when listening to your favourite music. I'm not going to reveal what I was listening to: I wonder if you can guess?

makeup

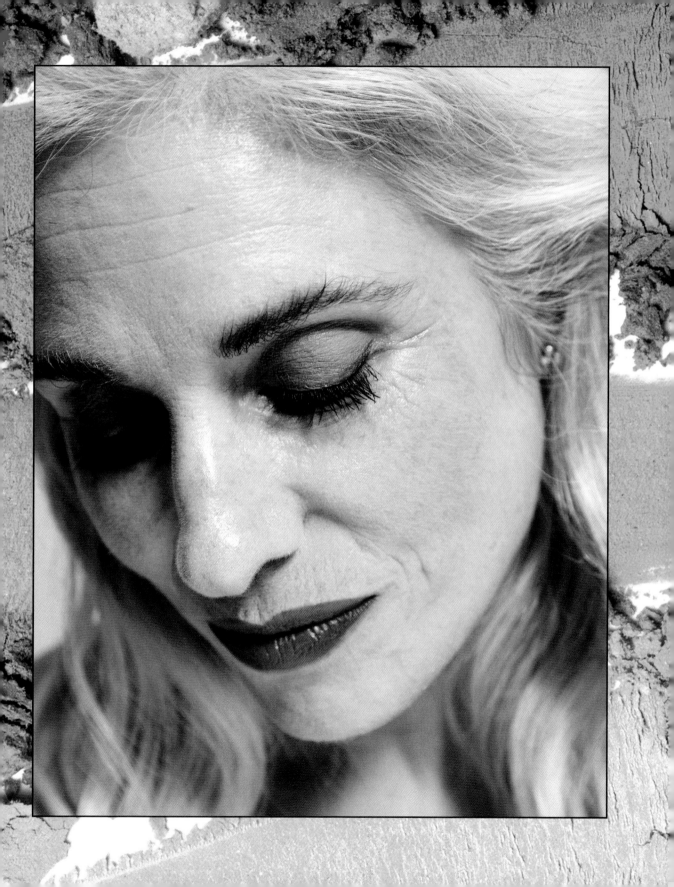

Here's how to create an editorial look based around these elements.

First prime the eyes with a cream-to-powder eyeshadow.

Define the eyes using a deep blue eye pencil and blend it out towards the socket using a small firm brush.

Pack aqua and teal eyeshadows onto the whole of the lid, using a fluffy brush to diffuse the colours, and apply a deep chartreuse colour towards the inner corner.

Use a small angled brush to pick up some of the black pigment from an eye pencil, and brush this softly along the upper lash line to define.

Curl the lashes and apply mascara to top and bottom lashes.

Apply foundation with a flat face brush, and use a smaller brush to apply concealer.

Line the lips with a pencil and apply some lip colour. Use the same lip colour on the cheeks for a subtle cohesive effect.

To complete the look, brush clear eyebrow gel upwards and outwards through the brows.

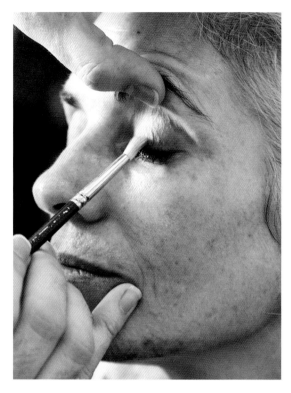

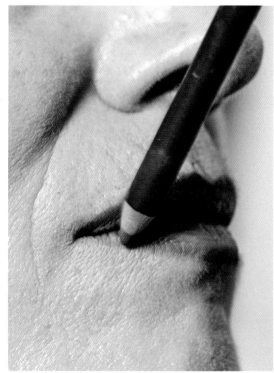

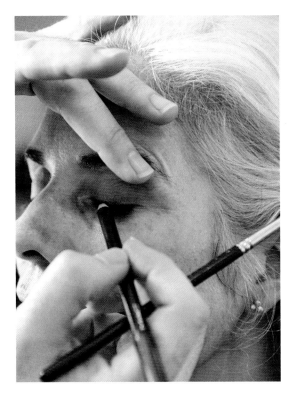

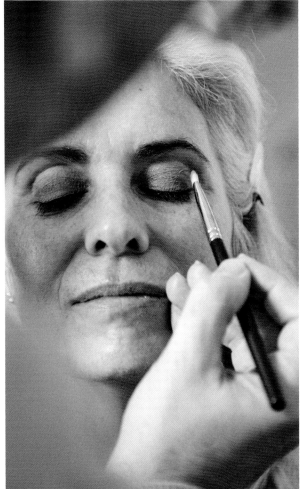

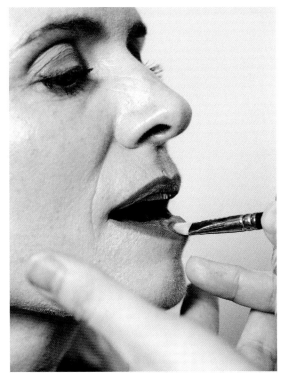

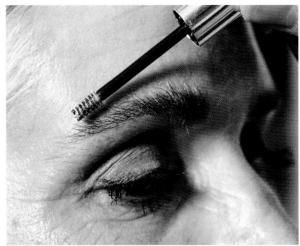

in the

I wish I had a penny for every time someone has asked me if I had got dressed in the dark. Well, now I can say that I've also painted a face in the dark! The idea behind this look is to see what happy little accidents can come out of doing makeup in the dark. During the experiment (p.90) I loved the weird use of purple and teal, and decided that they would be my focus for the editorial look. Here were two colours that I wouldn't have ever naturally put together, but suddenly fell in love with. When doing the experiment, I genuinely didn't have a clue what I was picking up or where it was going. I had tried to feel around to find features, but being blindfolded is so disorientating, and when I went to place gold leaf on the cheek bone it ended up hitting the jawline. I loved this too, along with the way the gold played off the colours. It made me think about how I could incorporate gold leaf into the eye area, but in a unconventional way. So I attached the gold leaf to the lashes with a little lash glue to secure it. This look ended up being rather club kid and chaotic, but there are elements that could be incorporated into many other looks and styles.

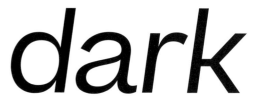

dark

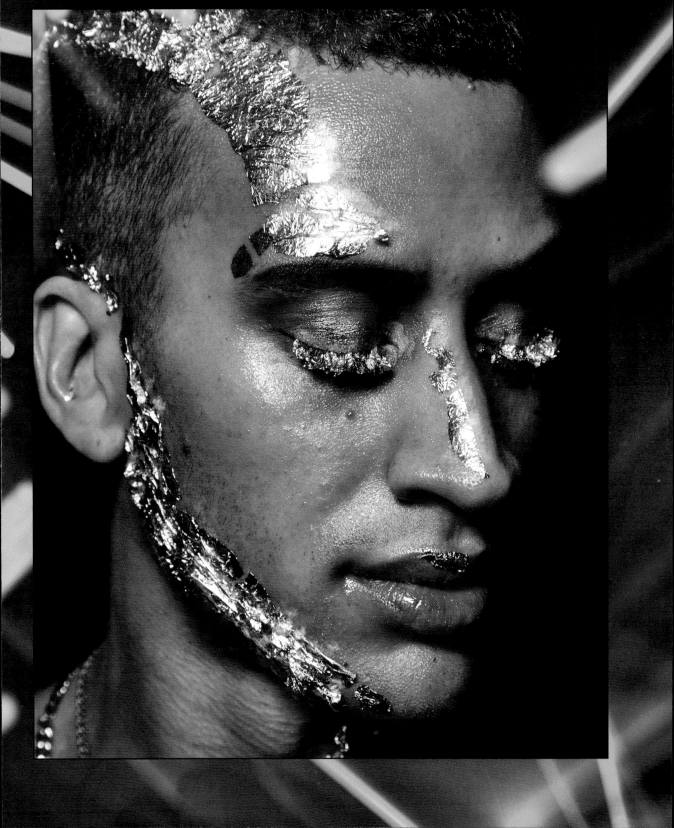

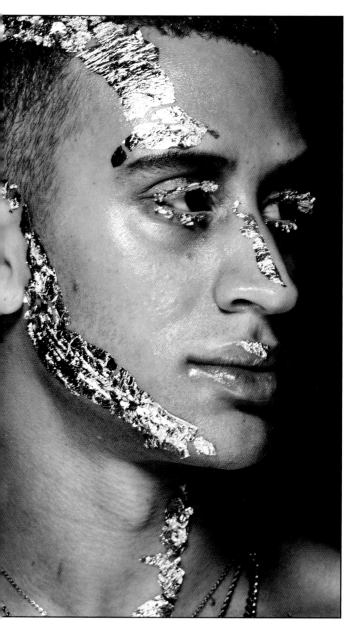

Here's how to create an editorial look based around these elements.

Curl the eyelashes and apply mascara. Using cotton swabs, place some gold glitter flakes on the eyelashes while the mascara is still wet so they will adhere. Build up the gold by applying more mascara and glitter flakes in the same way.

Use a small brush to pack teal shadow onto the top and bottom lash line. Blend it up towards the brow but leave the centre of the eyelid nude. Keep the colour more concentrated along the lash line and the inner eye.

After applying a moisturising balm over the face to make the skin glow and become tacky, place larger pieces of the gold leaf along the jawline, at the temple and down one side of the nose bridge.

Use a fluffy brush to pick up some shimmery gold powder and brush it over the lip and onto the centre of the eyelids, dusting it lightly over the high point of the cheekbones.

Dispense a little lip gloss onto the back of your hand then use a finger to dab it onto the lips and eyelids. Place some smaller gold fragments onto the cupid's bow and the neck.

Tightline the eyes using pale purple eyeliner pencil and apply a bluey-purple cream to the inner corner and over the lash line. Sweep a complimentary lilac to key areas and highpoints of the face like above the brow, cheek, chin and ear.

To finish, lightly mist with a setting spray to help the gold leaf stay in place.

DOM SAYS

IF YOU WANT GOLD LEAF TO LIE FLAT, GENTLY LAY IT DOWN AND THEN USE A SOFT, CLEAN BRUSH TO SMOOTH THE GOLD LEAF ONTO THE SKIN.

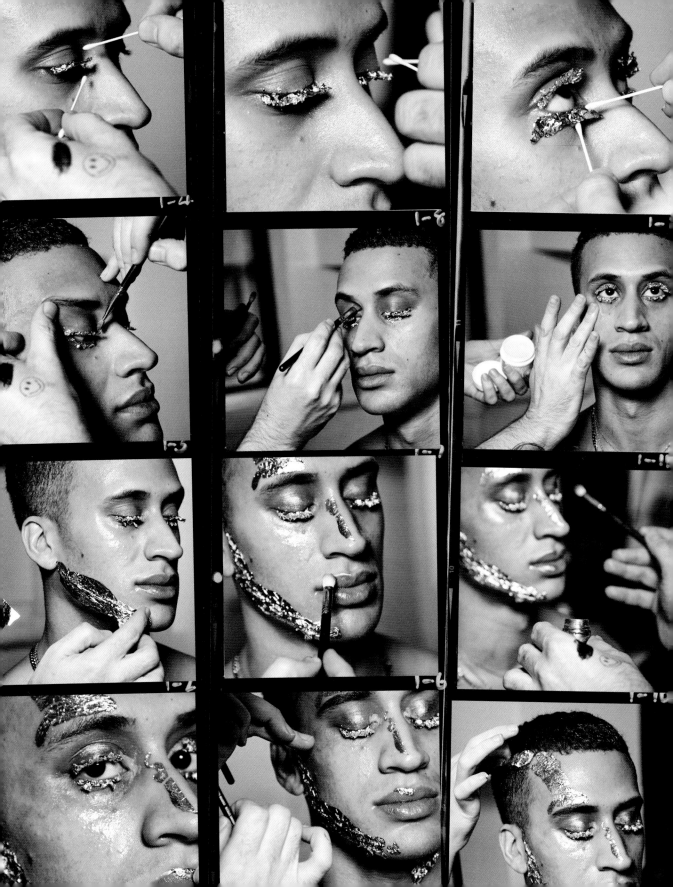

thanks

for

the

I'll let you in on a secret that I didn't reveal in the experiment (p.96): this model is my mum! The person who started it all, with me and makeup. I would sit and watch her apply it all the time, especially when she was going somewhere special, as that's when she would really go to town. One of my earliest memories is watching Mum paint her face, so it was a real honour to have her model for me: a full-circle moment. It was also only right, as the object I was using for the challenge was the clock her father built while she spent time building memories with him. I'll also let you in on another secret: Mum had no idea she was going to be a model for this book. I lured her to the studio on the pretence that she would watch the shoot, then told her one of the models hadn't turned up and she would need to step in. I'd like to say there was resistance, but Mum, ever the diva, took it in her stride. For this look, I worked with the rich, warm wood tones and the deep, tarnished gold and brass colours of the clock face and mechanism. These are not the usual shades my mum would wear, but I wanted to show how anyone can wear anything. I love this image. It's a memory of the day, as well as the collective memories of our pasts, and one I'll treasure in the future.
Thanks, Mum xx.

memories

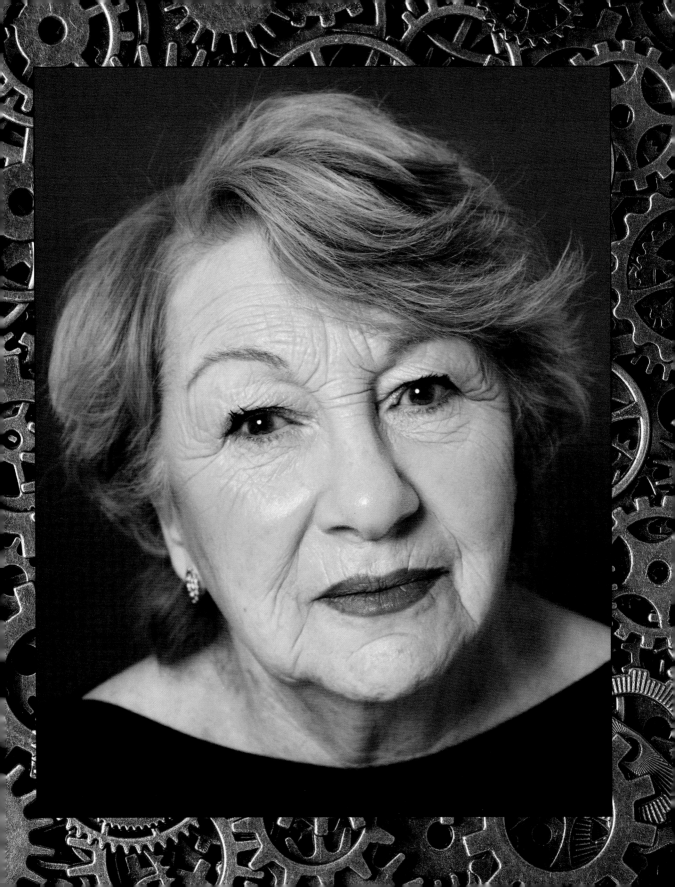

Here's how to create an editorial look based around these elements.

Prime and hydrate the face.

Starting with the eyes, line the upper lash line with a bronze eyeliner pencil and soften the line with a finger.

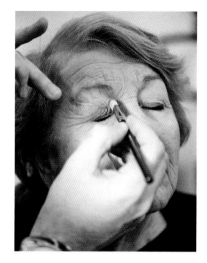

Brush a warm cream-to-powder eyeshadow over the entire lid.

Taking three shades of brown eyeshadow, apply these to the eyelid from lightest to darkest, working from the inner corner to the outer edge.

Add a shimmery gold to the centre of the lid and finish with two coats of mascara.

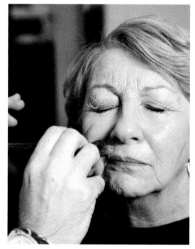

Dispense foundation onto the back of the hand then apply with a medium fluffy brush in circular motions using short strokes.

Line the lips with a light brown pencil and apply a rosy brown lipstick all over.

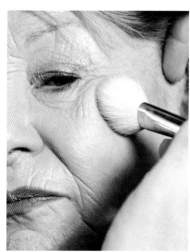

For an extra glow, add a warm blush with a fluffy brush to the cheeks, and cream highlighter to where light naturally hits the face.

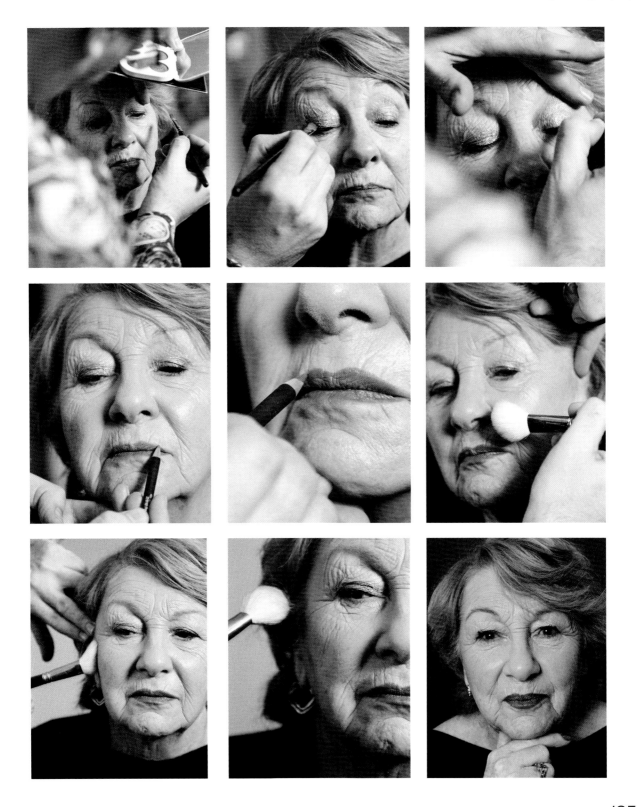

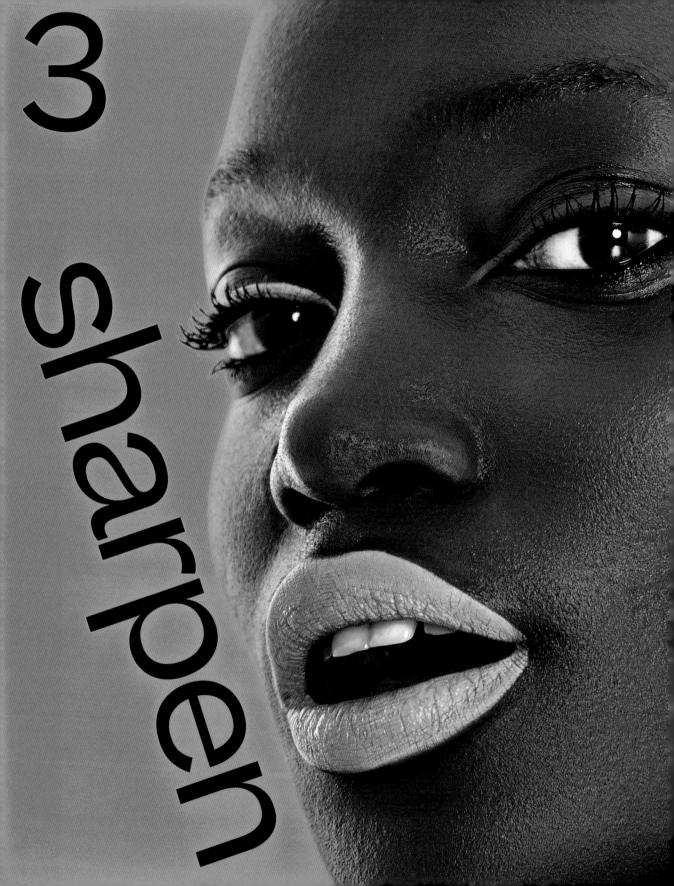

3

sharpen

your

skills

There are a thousand ways to slice an apple. Although there are some key techniques that will help you to achieve your desired look, I want to reiterate that we are all different. We all have our own way of holding brushes, and apply different amounts of pressure; we don't all use the same products, and certainly we are applying them to different faces. So, when asked for tips and tricks for perfecting makeup skills, which I very often am, it's not as straight forward as people would hope.

What I aim to provide within this chapter are the fundamentals to assist you with developing your own creative makeup style and individual expression. These basics will give you a starting point to help build your makeup repertoire, from helping you work out placements that suit you and your eye shape to tips on becoming a cosmetic mixologist. Some might seem obvious, such as defining a lip, others more obscure, like applying freckles, but all are here to help you start seeing what you could achieve, with just a little of the imagination and creative thinking you've gained from the previous chapters.

There are many places where you can go in order to gain basic knowledge of how to apply certain makeup techniques. But it's important to resist falling into the trap of being told what to do, of slavishly following someone else's routine. This section of Glowography is designed as an extension of the experiment and development chapters, enabling self-learning and new discoveries. Many techniques follow on from the looks created in chapter two, and will help you to refine your ideas into a single statement or concept, harnessing your creative flow in a more streamlined way.

Where most books work on the principle of starting with the basics and building up, I find that never really works due to the confinement and control it creates, instantly squashing any creative potential. I wanted my book to fling the doors of creativity wide open first, allowing you to just play and exercise the creative muscles that we barely get a chance to use. Once these muscles are strong, you can start training them to control the force of the creative explosion and hone your application to achieve your vision. In this chapter you will find tips to elevate your looks by fine-tuning symmetry, blending, precision and placement; you can also find tricks for making your look a bit more lived-in and undone, for no one wants perfection all the time, and who's to say what perfection is, anyway?

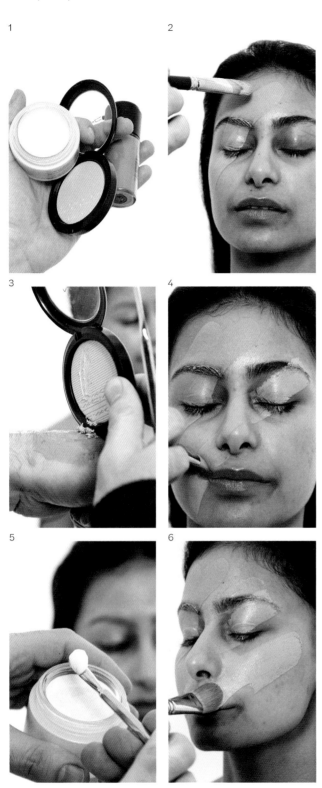

foundation manupulation

Most people don't realise that the formula of makeup can be easily altered using things you probably already have in your kit. Foundation especially can be changed to suit how you want your skin to look on any occasion.

Step by Step:

1, 2 Start with a matte liquid foundation: this can be made into more of a dewy or shiny base, but the opposite is not true – a dewy foundation can't really go matte without applying powder over the top.

3, 4 For an iridescent or glowy foundation, scrape some highlighter powder onto the back of the hand and mix with a pump of the matte liquid foundation.

5, 6 For a more radiant or dewy foundation, take a scoop of rich moisturiser and mix it with a pump of matte foundation.

Look around for other things you could mix in to change it up: a bronzer can deepen the shade for use when you want to warm up your complexion; a facial oil can produce a spa-like finish; or try adding some sparkly eyeshadow to shine like a star.

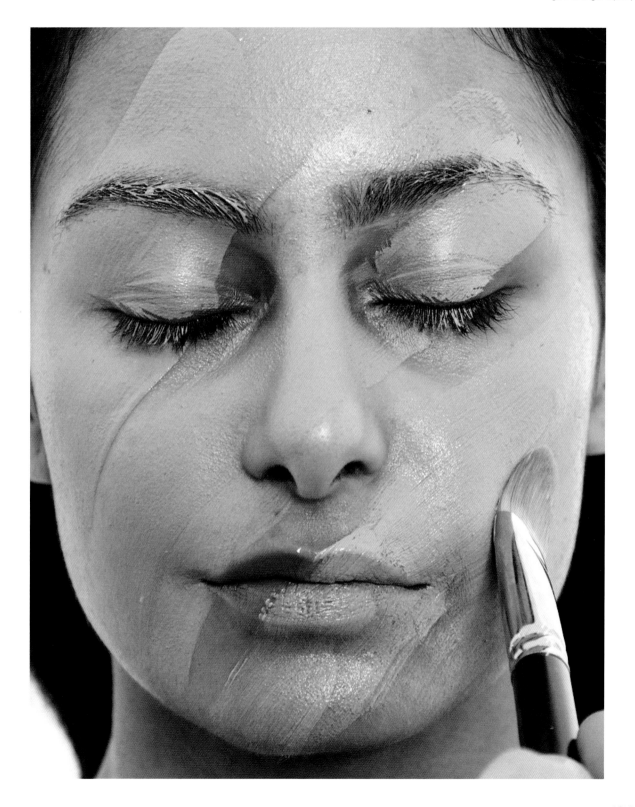

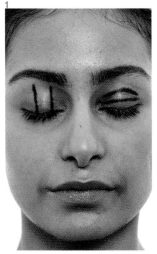

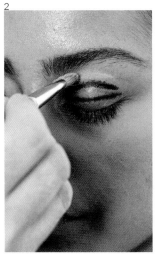

div-eye-d

There are no hard and fast rules with makeup, but there are some guidelines that can help you to master it. Consider placement: applying eyeshadow might seem straight forward, you just sweep it over the eye, right? But what if I told you your eye has natural divisions, and if you follow these you can never go wrong with your application. When applying eye makeup using more than one colour, simply break the eye down into thirds, either horizontally or vertically.

Step by Step

1   To do this horizontally, the eye already has two lines in place to help you. There is the socket, and between the socket and the lash line there's the crease, where the eyelid folds in on itself. To divide the eye up vertically, look in the mirror and draw two lines either side of your iris. This will give you three zones: outer, middle and inner.

2   For the horizontal divisions, place a light colour in the area above the socket line, a medium shade in the area in the middle (between the socket and the crease), and a dark colour between the crease and the lash line.

3   For the vertical divisions, do the same as you did on the horizontal eye, placing a light shade in the inner area, a medium shade in the middle and a darker shade in the outer area.

4   Pre-blending, you can see three disctinct bands of colour on both eyelids. When you do it for real you obviously won't have the guidelines.

5   Blend the shades together where they meet (see opposite).

Try swapping where you put the light, medium and dark shades. Different combinations will achieve varying results which will suit particular eye shapes. Play around and find the one that best suits you.

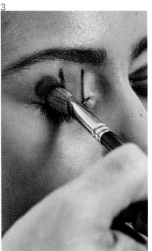

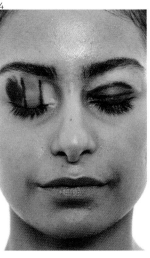

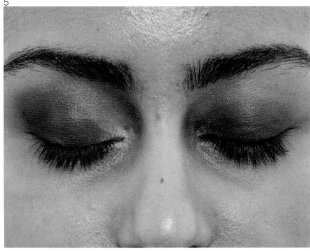

simple colour eye

To begin with the basics might seem a bit, well, basic, but mastering these will help you to unlock a whole new world of possibilities. Blending two colours together to create a seamless transition between them is the start of literally boundless makeup combinations.

Step by Step

1, 2 Prime the eye with a cream-to-powder eyeshadow or primer.

3 Using a small flat brush, apply one colour to the inner corner of the eyelid and blend towards the middle. Wipe off any excess from the brush and apply a new colour, this time working from the outer corner towards the centre of the lid.

4 Take a small fluffy brush and work the brush back and forth outside of the first colour to slowly soften the edge. Bring a fluffy brush to the middle of the eye and, moving it from side to side, work the brush from the lash line up towards the socket.

5 Remove any excess colour with a tissue, and work the same fluffy brush along the outside edge of the outer colour. However, instead of working it back and forth, make little circular motions as you go and note how the soft edge becomes more blended, with a greater gradient and fade out.

6 Blending colours together in this way gives you a seamless transition, which is endlessly versatile.

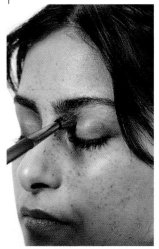

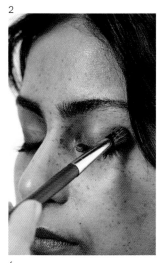

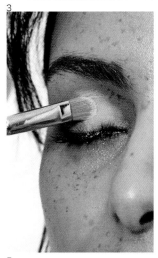

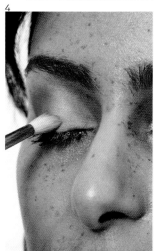

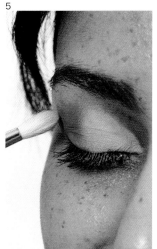

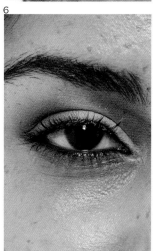

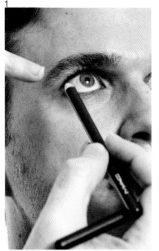

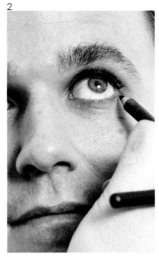

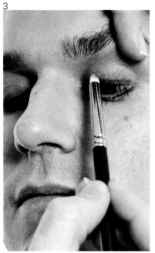

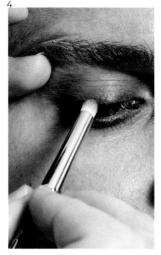

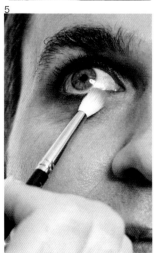

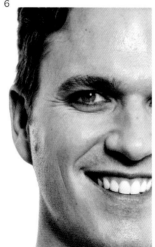

simple smoky eye

This simple but effective smoky eye was one of the first I learnt how to do. It is perfect for all eye shapes including individuals with a 'hooded' eye shape. Its nothing to do with carving out sockets but about elongating the eye.

Step by Step

1   Using an eyeliner pencil, draw a line along the top lash line.

2   Apply the pencil to the bottom lash line but not the waterline, and focus more on the outer corner.

3   Take a small eyeshadow brush and blend out the top lash line.

4   Use the eyeshadow brush or your finger to blend the bottom lash line out. For greater intensity, repeat steps 1–4.

5   Sweep a neutral brown eyeshadow over the lid and around the lash line from lash line to socket with a fluffy eyeshadow brush.

6   To finish, brush through the socket with any remaining shadow that's left on the brush. Run the brush along the smudged-out pencil of the bottom liner.

smudgy smoky eye

Makeup doesn't have to be complex and overly technical. It can be speedy and simple too. One of the earliest smoky eyes I learnt to do is this one and I continue to pull it out of the bag whenever time is tight.

Step by Step

1, Take a black or dark eye pencil and apply it quickly and messily to the upper and lower waterline. Load it up by layering it a few times.

2   If you find this difficult, try placing the end of the pencil near the inner corner of the eye and close your eye before pulling the pencil from corner to corner.

3   Once the waterline is loaded, close your eyes as tightly as possible and use your thumbs to rub across your eyes.

4   Open your eyes and you'll see that the pencil has smudged onto the eyelid and under the eye.

5   Use your finger to blend the smudge out to create a super-fast undone smoky eye.

6   Add a little iridescent shadow to the lid with your finger to really glam it up.

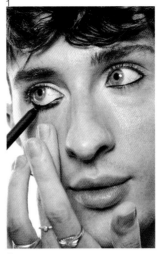
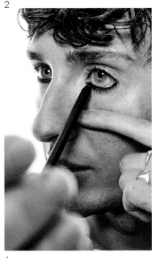
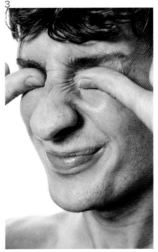
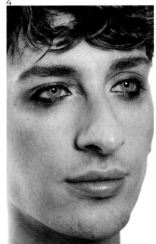
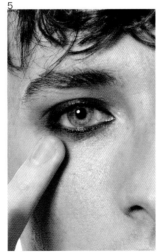
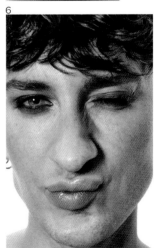

three-pencil smoky eye

You can 'smoke' anything out, including eye pencil. While rushing to get a client red-carpet ready one time, I created this smoky eye in just a few minutes in the back of a car as we were driving to the event. This look follows the same principles as the Simple Smoky Eye (p.194), but uses three eye pencils and works out and up instead of out and across.

Step by Step

1 Apply a light brown or gold eye pencil all over the lid and up into the natural socket.

2 Use a fingertip or small fluffy brush to smooth this out, blending up towards the brow bone.

3 Take the medium toned eye pencil and apply it over the eyelid, starting along the lash line and working up towards the crease of the lid.

4 Blend over the top with the fluffy brush, gently nudging towards the natural socket.

5 Apply the darkest pencil to the upper and lower waterline and along the lash line.

6 Use the fluffy brush to sweep over the darkest pencil, blending it into the medium brown shade.

7 Sweep under the eye with the brush as close to the waterline as you can to coax the darker shade from the waterline and out onto the skin. This gives a soft edge all the way around the eye.

8 To prevent the smoky eye from getting too big and out of control, sweep some face powder under the brow bone to soften the edge of the smoke and to stop it hitting the brow itself.

For extra glam, use a finger to lightly press some sparkly shadow over the lid, starting in the centre and gently tapping around.

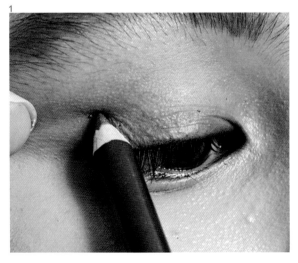
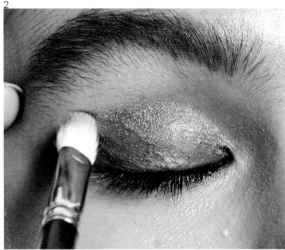

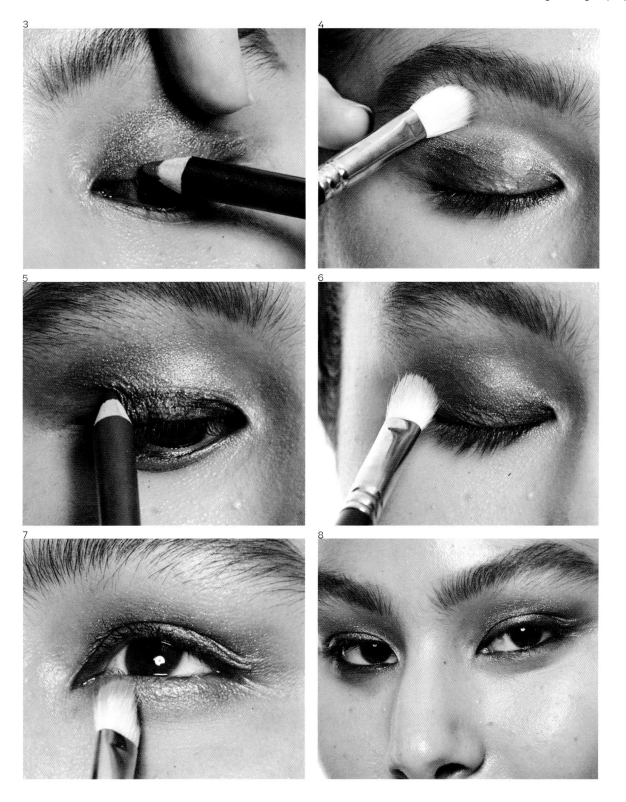

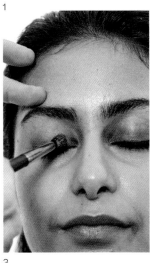

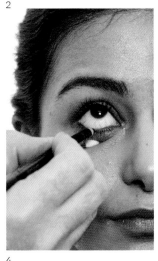

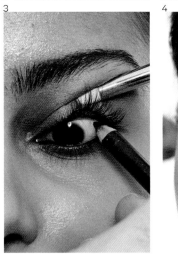

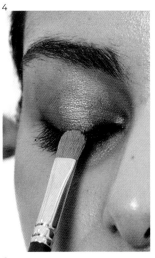

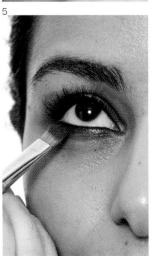

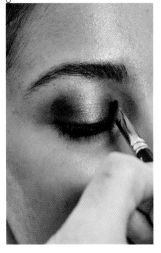

spot light smoky eye

This may seem like a more advanced style of smoky eye, but the principles are the same. The only difference is the placement. The beauty of this style is that you can easily adapt it to your unique eye shape.

Step by Step

1   Prime the eye with a neutral cream-to-powder eyeshadow or primer.

2   Apply a black or dark eye pencil to the waterline.

3   Use the same pencil along the upper and lower lash line, and soften it with a short firm brush.

4   With a small fluffy brush, apply a light shadow to the centre of the lid from lash to brow and then under the full length of the brow.

5   Use a firm flat brush to place a mid-tone shadow at the inner and outer corners of the eye, and sweep in towards the centre using the widest part of the brush. Mirror this under the eye using the thinnest part of the brush.

6   With the small fluffy brush, work over the edges of the mid-tone shade to soften them using circular movements.

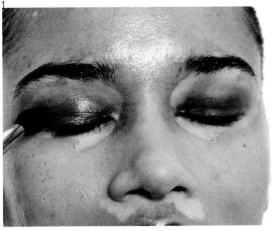

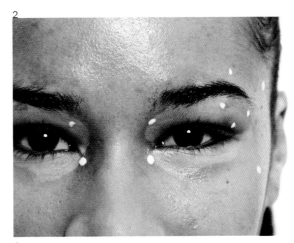

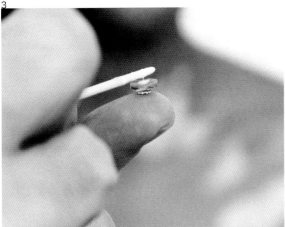

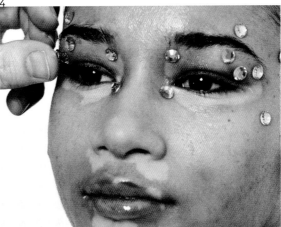

adornment eye

Adorning any look can add a fun and whimsical flare. Although gems and sequins are an obvious choice, this technique can be used to adhere anything to the skin. The placement doesn't have to be symmetrical but if you want symmetry, try doing each adornment one at a time, starting with non dominant side first. This will be the side in which you wouldn't normally start with.

Step by Step:

1   Apply any combination of eyeshadow in any style.

2   Dab lash glue in small dots around the eyes using a cotton swab. Place them between crease and brow, above the brow, around the temples and on the cheekbones.

3   Now apply lash glue to the backs of the gemstones and let the glue dry until it becomes tacky.

4   Stick these gemstones onto the positioned dots of lash glue on the face and press firmly to bond the glue. Lash glue works best when it's stuck onto itself rather than directly on the skin.

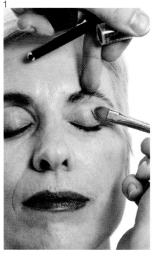

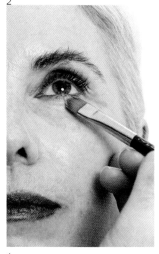

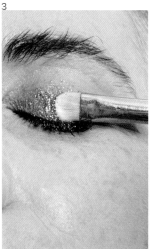

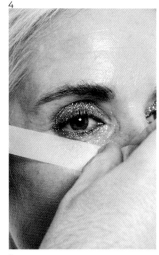

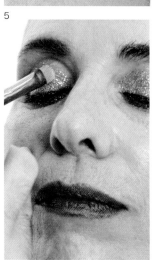

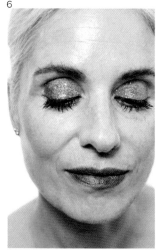

glitter eye

Glitter is always fun. Day or night, it can add a playfulness to your makeup as well as your personality. With this technique, you don't need to cover the entire eye lid, you could just add a little glitter to any of the other techniques in this section.

Step by Step

1   Dispense your chosen tacky product onto the back of your hand and apply it over the lid with a brush, from the lash line up to the socket.

2   Using the same brush, apply the adhesive along the bottom lash line.

3   Now pick up some cosmetic grade glitter using a flat eyeshadow brush, and apply it on top of the adhesive base, starting at the lash line. Press the glitter into the lid and then tap up and out.

4   Also press the glitter along the bottom lash line. Clean up any fallout using tape.

5   Repeat steps 3 & 4 using a lighter shade, but in a smaller and tighter area within the mid-tone colour.

6   Finish off with two good coats of mascara and softly sweep a little of the mid-tone shade through the socket of the eye. Place a touch of the lightest shade in the centre of the lower lash line.

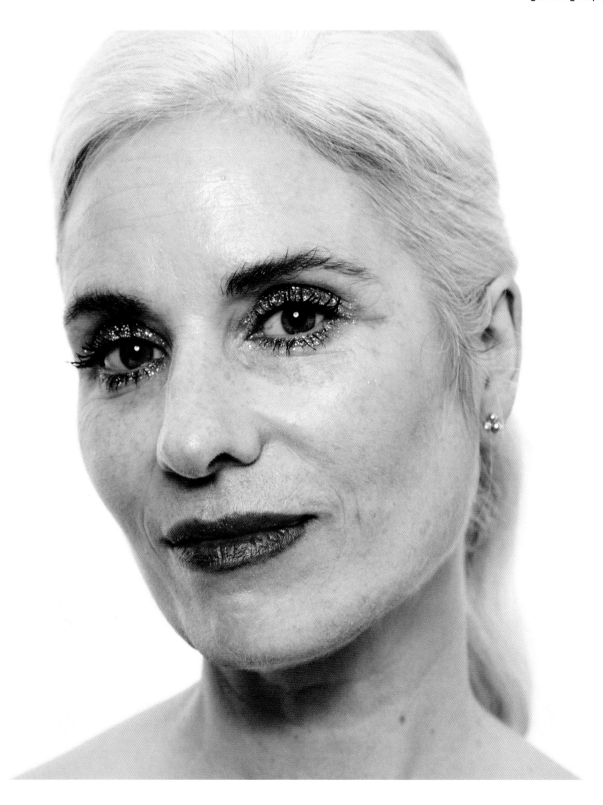

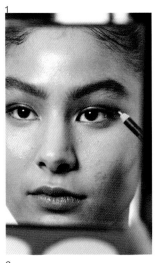

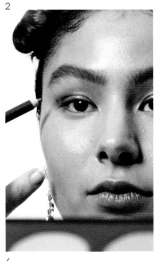

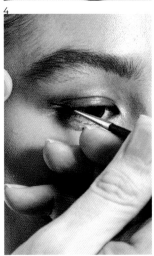

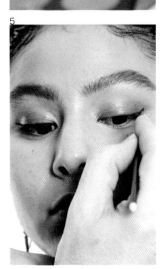

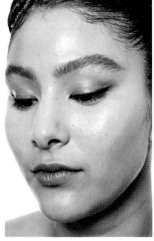

simple symmetrical eyeliner

I get asked how to achieve symmetry more than any other question. The key to symmetry is really looking. Our eyes will tell us if it's right. We often find fault when looking in the mirror, but you cannot put yourself down, you know: it's about focus.

Step by Step

Look at your eyes in the mirror and stare at your eyes. Imagine what and where the eyeline shoud be.

1   The best way to get symmetry is work on the eye, or side, that you wouldn't naturally start on. This is called the 'uncomfortable eye' because it's not so easy to work on. However, by focusing on the 'uncomfortable' eye first, you will find it easier to match it on the 'comfortable' or easier eye. With all this in mind, keep both eyes open and use a light colour pencil to draw a dot on your 'uncomfortable' side where you would like the eye liner to start from.

2   While still looking in the mirror, place a dot in the same place but on the more 'comfortable' side.

3   Check the dots are symmetrical. If not, only remove the dot from the comfortable side, and redo it.

4   Repeat steps 1-3 slowly building the line up to your desired shape.

5   Once you are happy with the placements, apply the line with a thin liner or angled brush. Begin at the dot and draw inward towards the centre of the lash line, keeping both eyes open as you go.

6   Repeat steps 4 & 5 on the opposite eye, keeping the eyes open. Once both are completed look to see if the eyes match. If not, remove and redo the easy eye until you are happy.

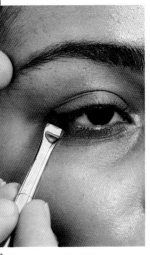
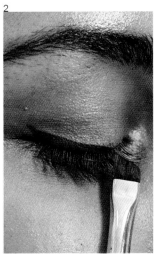

classic eyeliner

Eyeliner is not really about defining the eye by drawing a line on the lid, it's actually an enhancement of the lashes which then defines the eye. This is why traditionally it should be thinner in the inner corner, getting thicker as the line makes its way towards the outer edge, giving the impression of thick and full lashes. This is why eyeliner is a key look for so many and why mastering a classic liner can open the door to all sorts of liner looks.

Step by Step

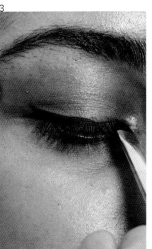
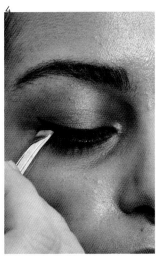

1   After loading a flat angle brush with product, place the short section of the brush to the outer end of the lash line and twist so that the longer section is pointing towards the end of the eyebrow. With the eye slightly open and looking straight ahead of you, draw in towards the centre of the lash line.

2   Fill in between the line and the lash.

3   Next, draw from the inner corner to the centre, with the longest part of the brush pointing towards the nose.

4   Repeat on the other eye.

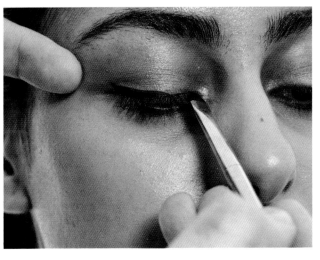

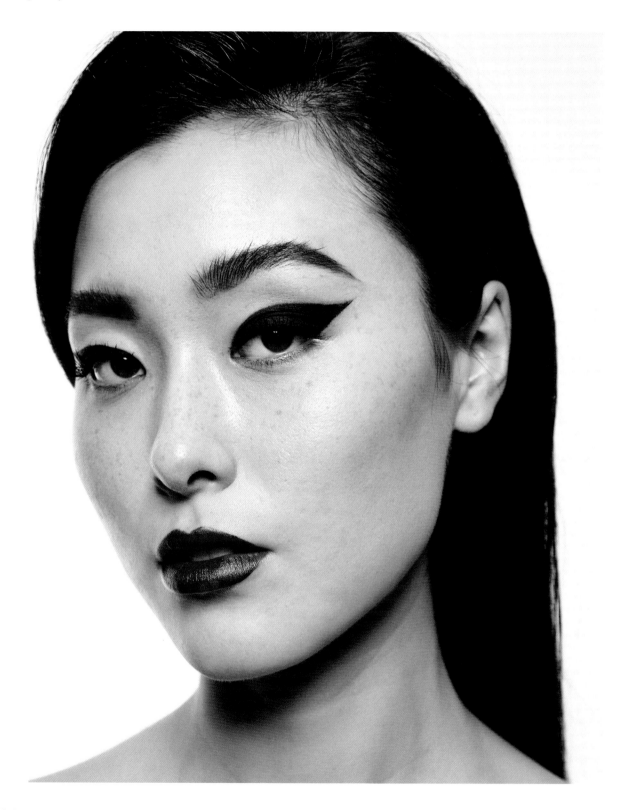

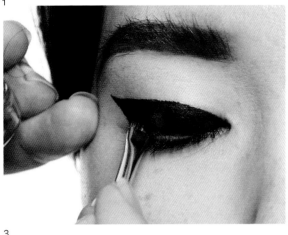

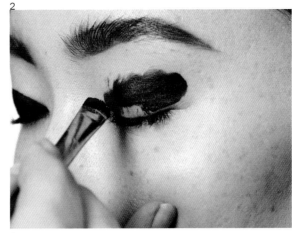

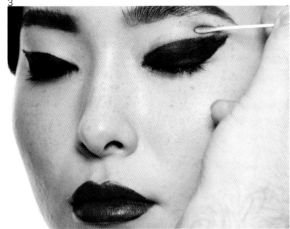

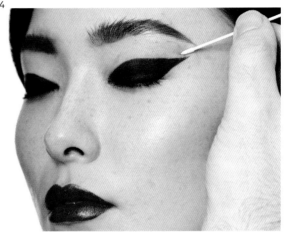

cut back eyeliner

Sometimes it's not what you add, it's what you take away. If I need to create a big, bold liner look, I will apply the desired line to one eye and then smother the other eye in a roughly applied line. Then it's all about chiselling away at the rough liner to work it back to the required shape.

Step by Step:

1   Using a flat, angled brush, pick up a little black eyeliner from a pot and line up the point of the brush to the end of the eyebrow, with the other end of the brush aligned with the outer edge of the lash line. With the eye slightly open, and looking down, draw in towards the centre of the eyelid. Next, draw from the inner corner to the centre, with the longest part of the brush pointing towards the nose. Fill in between the line and the lash.

2   Repeat on the other eye, but this time applying the eyeliner roughly, smothering it in a similar shape.

3, 4   With cotton buds and makeup remover chisel away at the rough liner to achieve the matching shape.

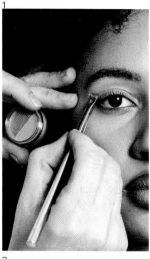

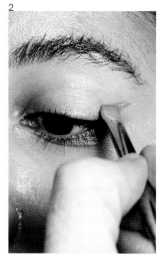

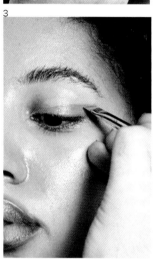

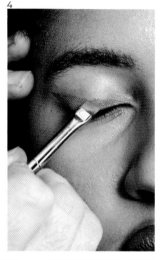

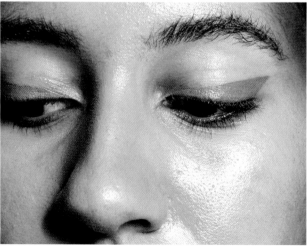

graphic liner

Nothing is more striking than a bold, strong and sharp eye line that, instead of enhancing your eye shape like the gentler classic eye liner, creates a more dramatic impression to the eye. A graphic eye line means business whether you are planning your next corporate takeover or popping to the shops because you've run out of biscuits.

Step by Step

1   With eyes looking directly into the mirror, place the flat edge of an angled liner brush to the outer edge of the eye with the end pointing up and out towards the end of the brow. Make a light mark with colour. A tip is to look at the swoop of the lower lash line from the inner corner, follow it down and then back up and continue out in the same direction.

2   Next, looking again into the mirror, press the edge of the angle brush from the crease line, straight out to meet the tip of the previous mark.

3   Follow this by using the flat side of the angle brush, loaded with colour, and press into the triangle shape you created, then sweep in towards the inner corner of the eye.

4   Finish by drawing from the inner corner of the eye up to meet the eye liner.

creative eyeliner

Now you've created a big bold graphic line, you might as well have some fun with it. Here I show you how a simple carry over from the printable experiment (pp.64 and 152) can create a fun and creative play on a graphic eye line.

Step by Step

Start by working through steps 1 to 4 from Graphic Liner (see opposite).

1   Take your printable item and paint it with a cream or gel-based eyeshadow or eyeliner.

2, 3   Press the painted item against the eye, starting on the outer edge.

4   Using a cotton swab and makeup remover, neaten the edges of your graphic liner for a sharper effect.

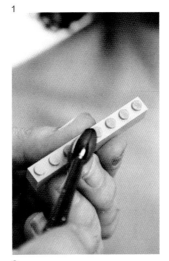
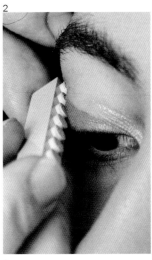
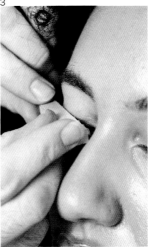
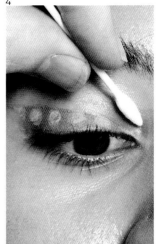
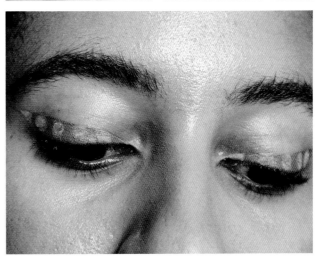

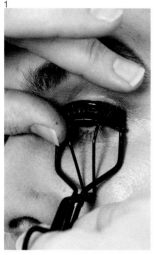

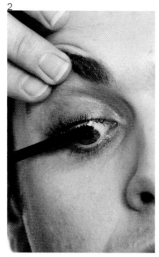

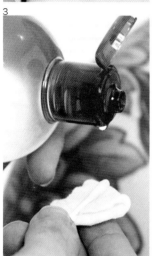

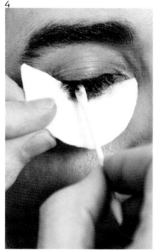

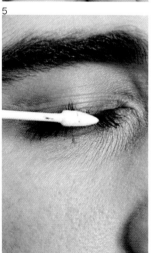

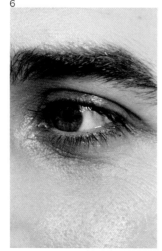

tinted lash mascara

The use of mascara to define the eyes is not a new thing; it can be traced back over 5000 years. But it doesn't have to just be used for a fluttery effect. A simple sheer wash of colour on the lashes can give a subtle definition that is not obvious but still effective in making your eyes strangely more captivating.

Step by Step

1   Always start by using an eyelash curler to lift the lashes.

2   Lightly apply a coat of mascara to the top lashes.

3   Fold a cotton pad in half and dampen a cotton swab with eye makeup remover.

4   Place the cotton pad beneath the lashes. Lower your lid, stroke the lashes from root to tip with the bud.

5   Use a dry cotton bud to achieve a natural-looking tint.

6   Curl the lashes once more to finish.

clumpy lash

Clumpy lashes are a fashion week staple because it's on the extreme side of definition. However, when used as part of an everyday look, it can add wonderful intensity while giving fashion when used with a paired back look.

Step by Step

1 First curl the lashes.

2 Apply one coat of mascara to the top lashes, beginning at the roots and making zigzag motions while brushing upwards.

3 Apply mascara to the bottom lashes, again working in zigzag motions from root to tip.

4 Moving the tip of the wand in circular motions, work another coat of mascara along the bottom lashes from the inner corner to the outer edge.

5 Repeat with the top lashes, working the wand from root to tip in the direction of the natural lashes to achieve a fan effect.

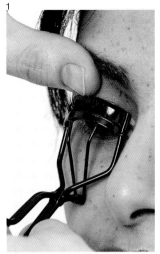
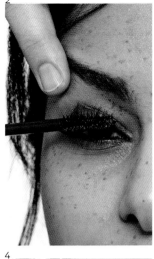
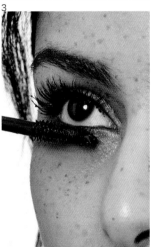
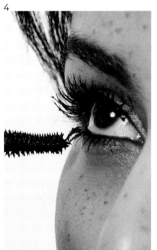
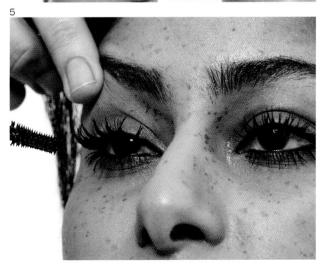

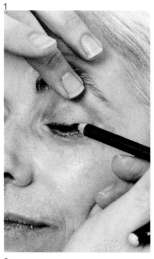
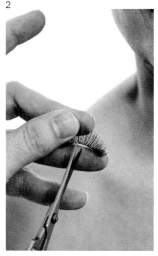
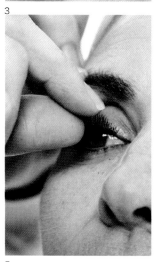
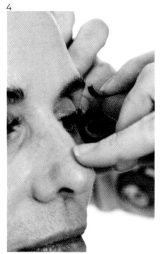
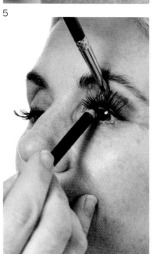
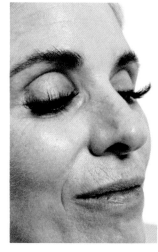

false lash made easy

False lashes have the unique ability to add instant glamour and drama to any look for any occasion, although they can bring many people out into a panic sweat. As someone who really struggled with applying lashes, I think this simple trick will help you master a false lash look without getting glue everywhere.

Step by Step

1   Start by applying a soft brown eye pencil to the top lash line, then use a pencil brush or your fingertip to smudge the pencil line out.

2   Take one of the lashes and cut it into equal thirds along the spine. Apply some lash glue to the spine of each of the lash sections and pop them back into the container, spine-up, to let them dry.

3   Starting with the middle lash section, gaze directly into a mirror with the head tilted back and place the lash over the centre of the eye, as close to the lash line as possible. Do the same with the other eye, checking in the mirror for symmetry.

4   Take the inner-third section and place it in the inner portion of the lid, leaving an approximate 2–3mm gap from the innermost corner. If this means that the two lash spines overlap slightly, that's fine. Do the same with the outer lash, leaving a couple of millimetres gap from the very outer edge, again allowing overlap with the lashes if there is any. Repeat for the other eye.

5   Fill in any gaps between the real lashes and false lashes with an eye pencil or deeper shade of eyeshadow, and apply mascara to blend.

bold false lash

A phrase I've always loved is 'Go Big or Go Home!' And sometimes I feel the same way about lashes. To apply lashes to the top and bottom lash line can look bold, but if you want to bring the drama there really is nothing better. The trick with all falses lash applications is to know that one eyelash is not going to wanna play. That way, when one does decide to not go in the right place first time you won't be frustrated, you'll simply peal it off and go again.

Step by Step

First apply the Classic Eye Liner (p.203).

1   Now apply black pencil in the lower waterline and smudge it out with a brush.

2   Remove the lashes from their container and place them loosely along the lash line. Ideally they should start and end a few millimetres outside of the inner and outer corner of the lash line. Cut the strip down to size if needed.

3   Paint lash glue onto the spine, and leave to dry fully.

4   Place the spine of the lashes over the liner as close to the natural lashes as possible, starting in the middle and then lightly pressing the outer and inner corners to the lash line. Repeat this process with the bottom lashes.

5   Apply a little mascara to help blend the false lashes with the real ones and to add extra drama.

6   Apply some dark powder in any areas of visible skin between the false and real lashes.

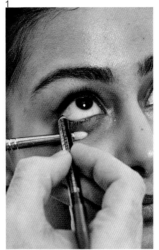
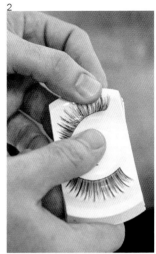
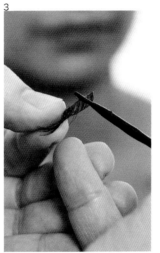
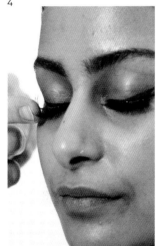
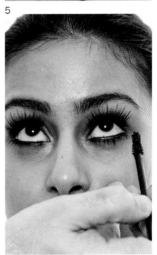
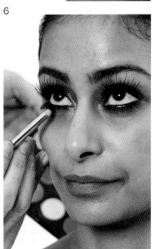

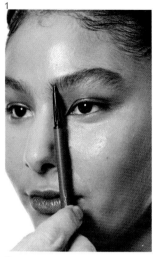

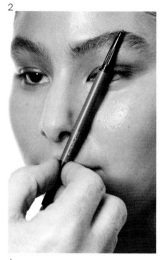

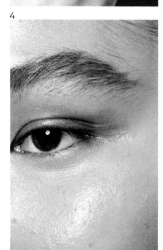

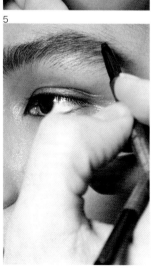

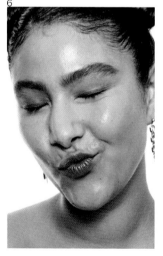

soft + natural brow

Never underestimate the power of a good brow. They may only be the support act to the rest of the makeup, but without them the look just doesn't feel complete. The first thing you need to understand about brows is how we view them. They are individual short hairs, true, but what we see is more than that. We see the shadow formed by the hair first, then we see the hair on top. So if you want to create a natural looking brow, the trick is to match the colour to the shadow of the brow and not to the hair itself.

Step by Step

1   Pick a brow pencil or powder colour that most closely matches the shadow of the brow, and hold either pencil or brush vertically from the nostril to the inner corner of the eye. Draw a dot where the tip of the pencil or brush meets the brow. This is where the brow should start.

2   Twist the tool to cross the pupil, with the end still held against the nostril, and place another dot just above the natural brow. This indicates the placement of the arch.

3   For the final dot, still keeping the bottom of the tool against the nostril, twist it some more to be in line with the outer corner of the eye and place a mark where the tip meets the brow.

4   Now that you know the shape of the brow, use small, short dashes in an up and out motion to draw in a straight line from the marker closest the nose to the one in the middle above the natural brow. Don't be tempted to go with the curve.

5   Continue the dash motion, but move to a horizontal direction as you go from the middle marker to the end of the brow.

6   If there are any gaps, apply a few dashes with a darker colour to mimic the natural hair.

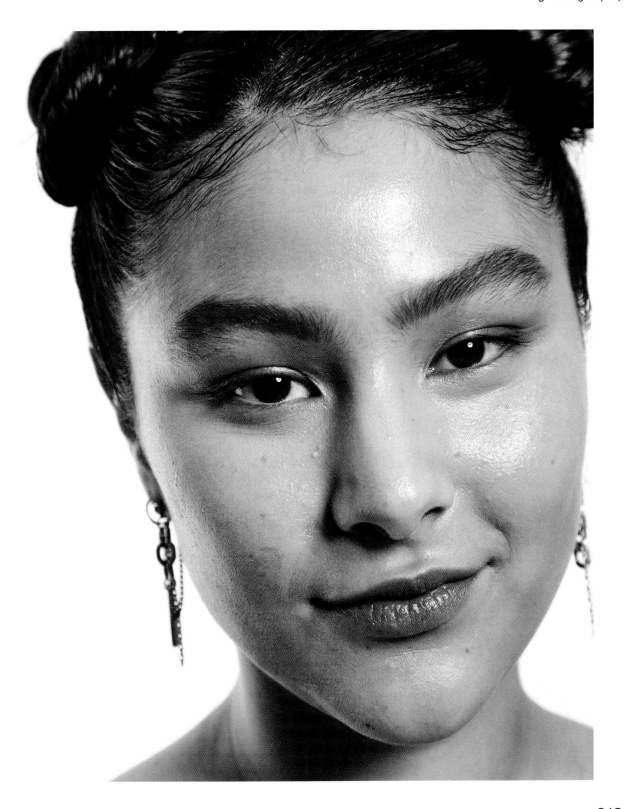

1

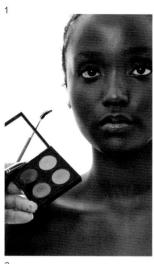

2

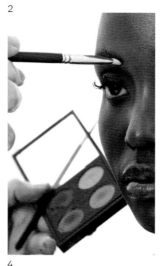

3

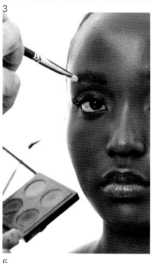

4

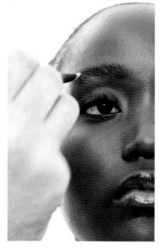

5

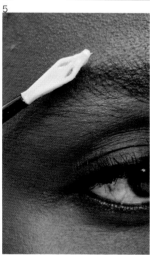

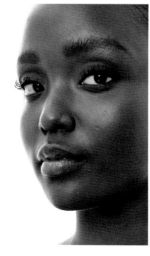

full + fluffy brow

One of my favourite brows to do is a brow that looks full and fluffy but natural at the same time. Most common during fashion week, it's a style that has started to cross over to the red carpet but not yet much to everyday wear.

Step by Step

1   Sticking with the basic shape created for the Soft Natural Brow (p.212), use a flat eyeshadow brush to pick up some colour that is one or two shades lighter than your natural brow.

2   Place the brush beneath where the brow starts, nearest to the nose, and brush up.

3   Continue brushing up from the bottom or base of the brow, moving slowly across the brow in a straight line up towards the natural arch.

4   Pick up some more colour and place the brush slightly above the natural arch, sweeping it down and across, just above where the natural brow grows. Once you've created the shape, work over the brow with more colour to create a full but soft appearance.

5   Use clear brow gel to brush the brows up, and only up, all along the shape so that the outer end of the brow is brushed and groomed into the shadow just beyond where the hair naturally grows.

strong + defined brow

In the beauty world, a pared-back makeup look with a strong and defined brow can be the last word in chic. It's not always about going dark, it's more about strength, sharpness and precision. Some people have trouble when they try to draw the curve into the brow – the key is to keep all the lines straight and let the curve of your face create the illusion of a curved brow.

Step by Step

1   Using the same shape as created for the Soft + Natural Brow (p.212), map out the placement for your strong brow.

2   Take a shade that is just slightly lighter than your natural brow, or a totally different colour altogether, and begin drawing a straight line along the bottom of your brow. Start from the inner corner closest the nose and move straight in the direction of the arch. This line is called the base line.

3   Once you've created this single straight line, continue it from the top of the arch down towards the tail of the brow, just beyond where the natural brow grows.

4   From this outer brow tip, draw a straight line along the bottom of the brow to meet the original base line.

5   From the top of the arch, draw one more straight line along the top of the brow towards the inner corner where you started. Keep it parallel to the original base line.

6   Now that you have a perfectly sharp and crisp outline, simply fill it with your chosen colour and clean up any edges with mini cotton swabs and foundation.

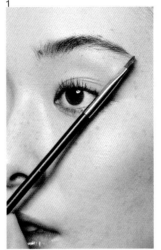
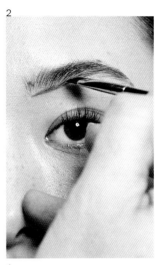
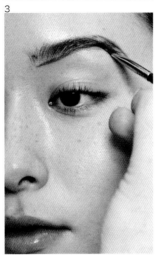
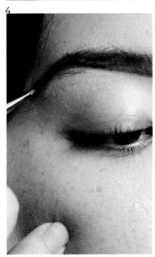
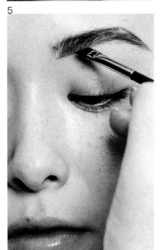
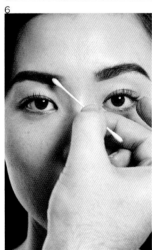

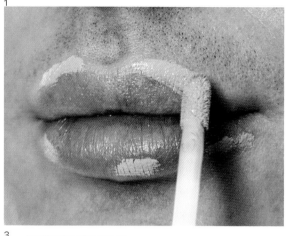

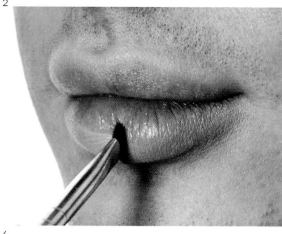

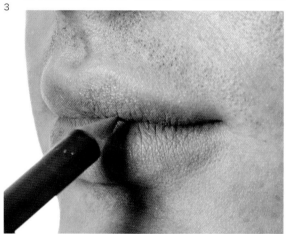

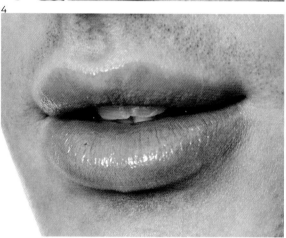

soft pout lip

This soft ombre lip is a go-to for anyone who doesn't necessarily feel comfortable or confident wearing a fuller lip. It's great for any occasion where you want to elevate your style without being too bold.

Step by Step:

1   Start by applying a little concealer to the lip line.

2   With a small flat lip brush, blend the concealer out.

3   Take a lip pencil and apply it to the centre of the lips, working out from where the lips meet towards the lightly applied concealer.

4   With a clean brush, apply your favourite lip balm over the lips to blend the pencil and concealer together.

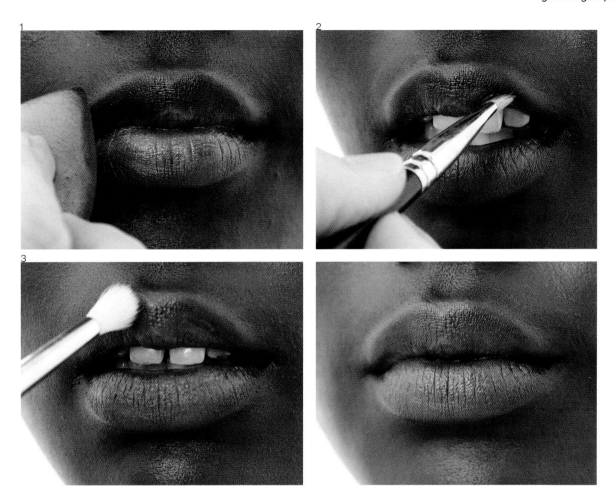

soft edge lip

Many people love the idea of wearing colour on their lips but either feel too self-conscious or uncomfortable wearing a fully loaded lip. Giving your lips a soft edge with concealer enables you to wear colour without it filling the entire lip.

Step by Step:

1   Use a beauty blender or a fluffy brush to buff a little concealer or foundation around the edge of the lips.

2   Apply your chosen lip colour to the centre of the lips with a small flat lip brush.Start working the colour out using short smooth strokes, but do not let it reach the edge of the natural lip outline.

3   Using a small fluffy brush, start brushing over the line where the lipstick meets the concealer to achieve a smooth and seamless blend.

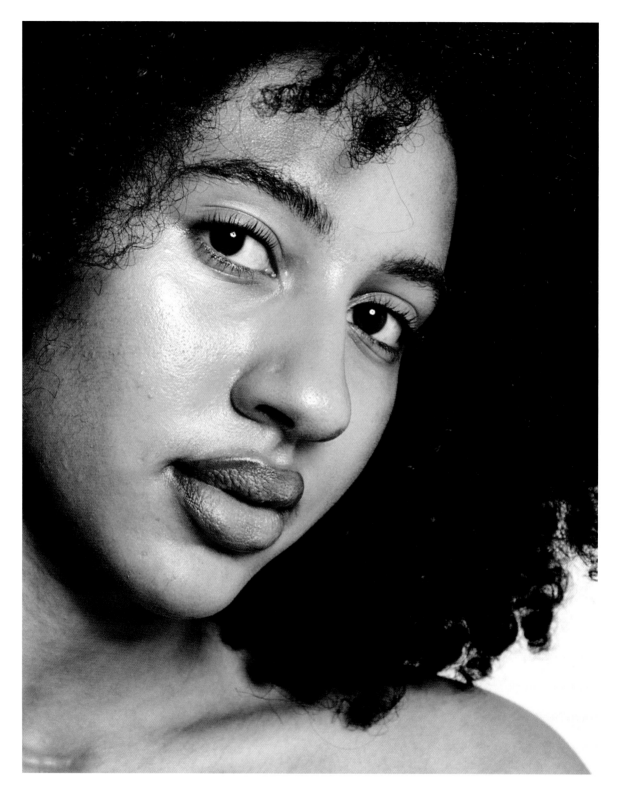

contoured lip

To achieve a fuller appearance to your lip you don't need to only look towards a medical procedure, you can use simple contouring and highlighting techniques to give the illusion of a plumper, poutier lip.

Step by Step:

1   Apply a lip colour that is a shade lighter than your natural lips.

2   Using a grey-toned lip pencil, draw along the lip line, letting it blend out of the lip shape and just beyond the natural lip line.

3   Using a small brush, blend out the lip line edge.

4   Now choose a darker brown lip pencil and draw along the natural lip line.

5   Blend the pencil into the lip and add more colour to the edges of the lip. Finally, take a lip brush and blend the darker lip liner into the pale lipstick.

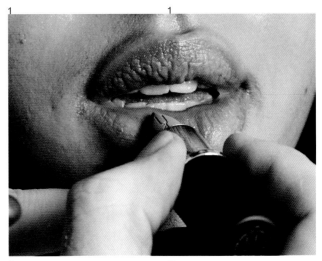

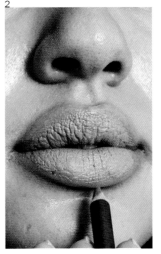

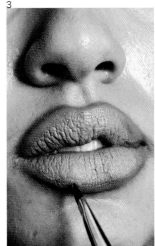

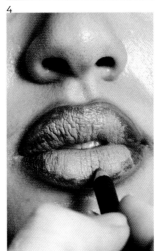

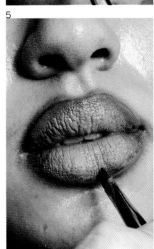

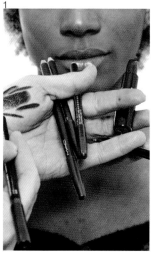
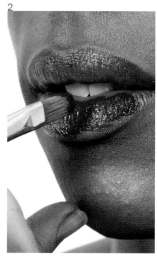
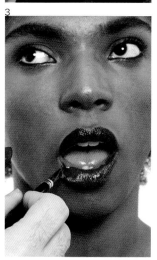
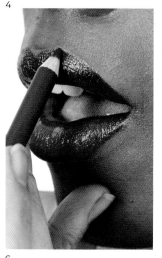
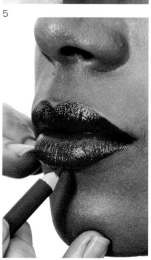
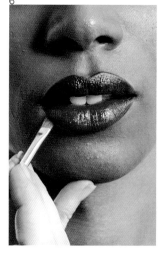

classic sharp lip

A staple of any MUA's repertoire is the ability to create a perfect red lip. However, it doesn't really matter what colour it is, the technique is still the same. A strong, bold, precise lip will always command attention, and if you can nail this, it means you can do anything.

Step by Step

1 Pair your lip colour to a matching lip pencil. This may take time to get right, but it's important to get it as close as possible.

2 Start by applying the lip colour – yes, the lip colour, not the lip pencil – to the centre of the lip with a small flat brush, and work slowly towards the lip edge. Starting with the lip colour means you're not wasting time trying to get the perfect outline. Fill it and move on.

3 Once the colour is on, look at the lip shape. It will now be easier to see what needs to be done in order to achieve a more symmetrical and balanced shape.

4 Using the lip pencil, start slowly drawing around the lip edge, lifting and filling the lip line where needed to get an even shape.

5 For balance, look at which lip is biggest (upper or lower) and use that as your guide to increase the size of the smaller lip.

6 If needed, apply a little concealer on an angled brush to sharpen and clean up the edges.

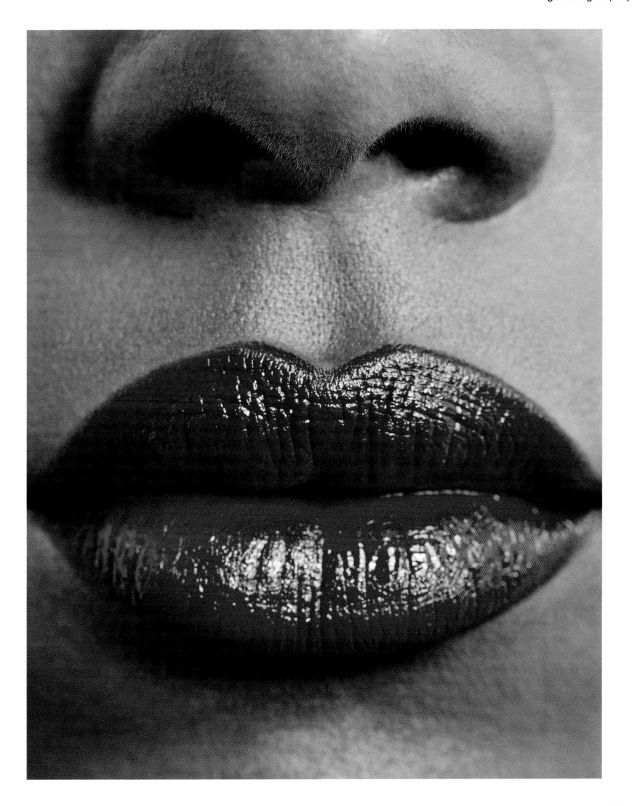

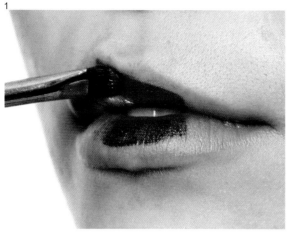

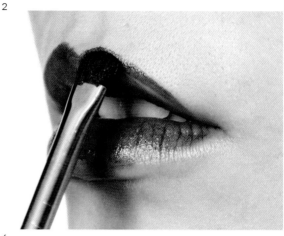

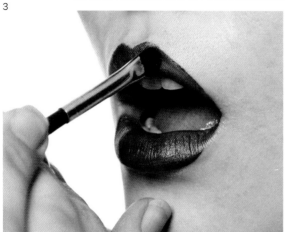

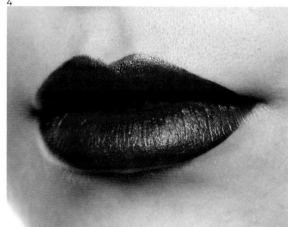

ombre lip

An ombre lip is a classic lip look for those who want to try something new. It's a relatively easy technique, however it can be challenging if you don't get the colours or tones right. Remember, it's far easier to start with a lighter shade and add something darker than it is to begin with a darker shade and try to make it lighter.

Step by Step:

1   Using a small flat brush, take a lighter coloured lip product and apply it to the majority of the lip, with the focus being on where you want the light to be most visible (i.e. the centre of the lip or the outer edge). Here the focus was the centre.

2   Take the darker or deeper colour on the same brush and apply it to the sections of the lip which have yet to see any colour.

3   Next, slowly blend the darker colour into the lighter one with the brush.

4   To make the light colour pop, add a little more if needed.

powder lip

A bright matte lip can really sing. The matte texture, though not reflecting light, still radiates with an intensity of colour. Topped with powder makeup, it can almost glow. This type of lip works perfectly with a softer or more subtle eye and should be regarded as a key accessory.

Step by Step

1   Apply your chosen colour with a brush and perfect the shape with a matching lip pencil mirroring the technique from p220.

2   Find a powder, either loose or pressed, that matches the shade and tone of your lipstick and load up a small flat applicator brush. Press the powder onto the lip starting on the bottom lip, placing a tissue under the lower lip to catch any fallout. Continue pressing the powder onto the bottom and upper lip using the tip of the brush against the outside of the lip.

3, 4   Use a cotton swab or a tissue dipped in makeup remover to clean up any messy edges or powder fallout.

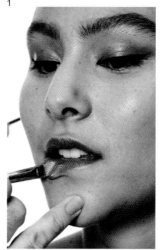
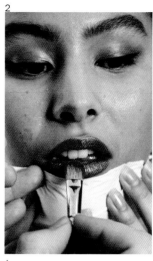
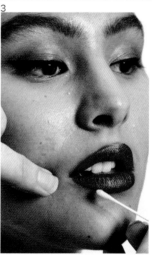
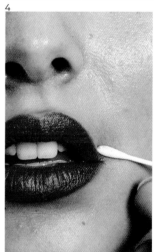
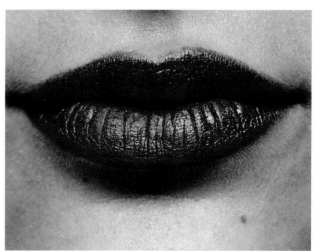

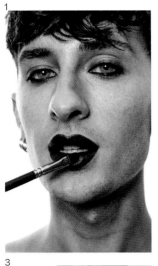

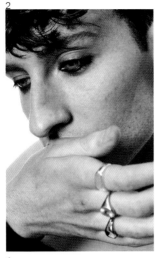

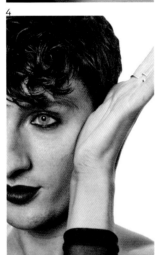

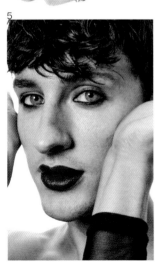

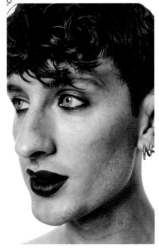

kiss it off blush

Makeup doesn't need to be laboured over it can be quick and speedy too. If time is short, this quick makeup hack is a great way to add colour to the cheeks while knowing it will compliment the lips. I've used this technique on many clients for many a red carpet rush while in the back of a cab on route to the event and no one is any the wiser.

Step by Step

1   Apply your lip colour as normal.

2   Kiss the heel of your palm.

3   Lace the fingers of both hands and rub the heels of your palms together.

4   Holding your hands up at either side of your face with palms facing out, place your thumbs on top of your ears.

5   Roll the heel of your palms down onto your cheeks repeatedly, moving towards your nostrils.

6   This gives an instant kiss of blush to match your lips, perfect every time.

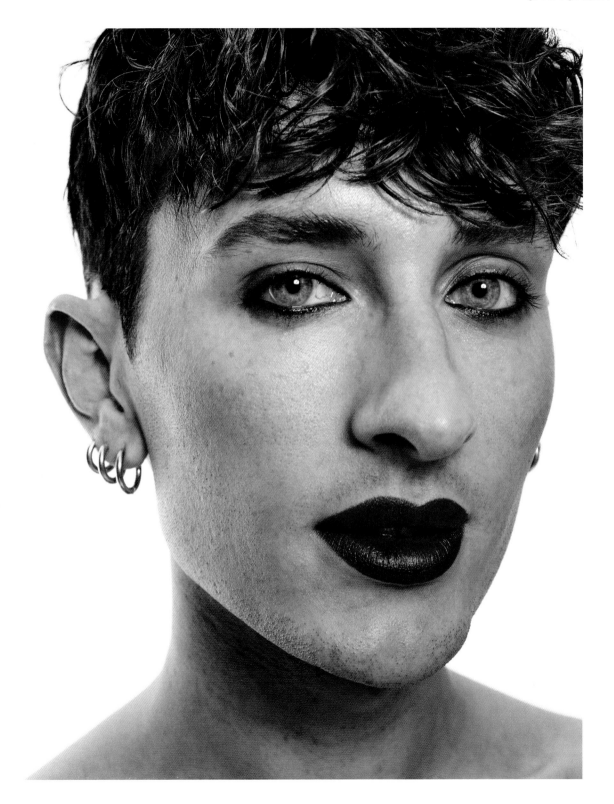

1

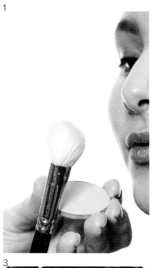

2

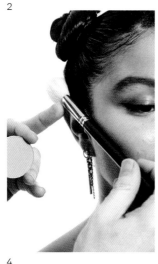

unfussed blush

Whenever I do a masterclass, I'm always amazed by how often the simplest things make the most impact. For instance, having only applied blusher one way during my entire career, I didn't realise that no one else did it the same way as me, that most people brush upwards. By 'blushing down', the colour ends up on the cheek and cheek bone, creating a much more flattering placement that colours and subtly contours at the same time.

Step by Step

1   Use a large fluffy brush to sweep over the blusher powder and tap off any excess.

2   Place the brush on the cheek bone, with one end above the ear and the other pointing towards the mouth. This is the placement and direction you should apply your blush.

3   In a straight line, pull the brush down towards the corner of the mouth without curving around the cheek. Let the brush flick away from the skin. Repeat this brushstroke three or four times.

4   Now change the direction of the stroke and brush down from the same starting point, but this time towards the bridge of the nose.

3

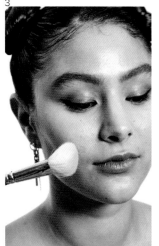

4

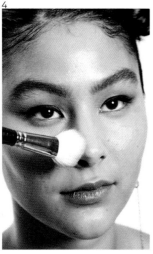

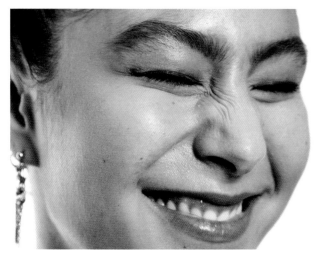

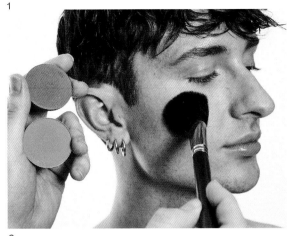

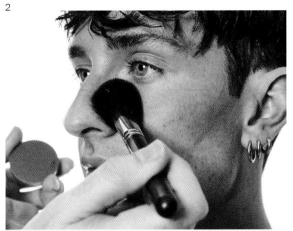

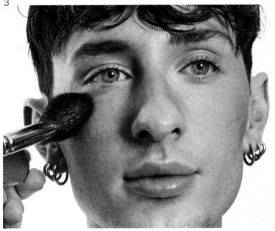

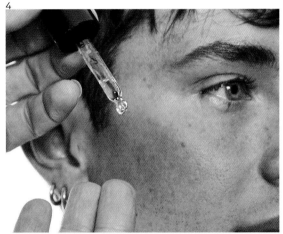

sun sweep blush

Blusher works on many emotional levels: it can be used to create a flirtatious flush, a youthful pinch, or a colourful pop to intensify the eye colour. It can also create a 'first days of summer' glow, and for this blush you'll need two shades, one that's hotter than the other, a more orange or red, and a large fluffy brush.

Step by Step:

1   Begin by applying the first, non-hot, shade of blush to the cheek, starting directly in line with the outer corner of the eye and sweeping down in a straight line towards the tip of the nose.

2   Next take the hotter shade of blush and, using the same fluffy brush, brush in a horizontal straight line from cheek to cheek, lightly dusting the bridge of the nose in between.

3   With whatever is left on the brush, sweep lightly left to right and up into the hair line.

4   For added heat, tap a little facial oil over the hotter shade of blush.

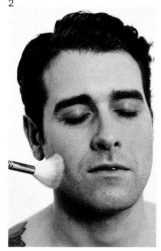

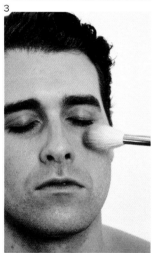

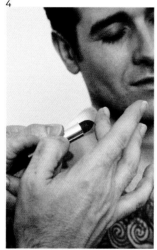

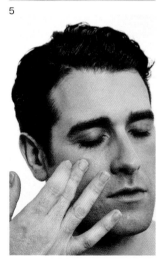

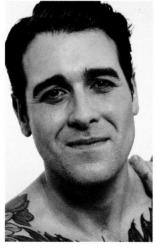

real bronzer

Bronzer is a staple for many people as it can revive the skin if you're maybe not feeling it. Most people apply their bronzer all over the face or just on the cheeks to warm the skin. However, if you treat the bronzer like sun and drape the colour over the skin in downward strokes it can look lived in and real as if you're on an endless vacation.

Step by Step

1   Stand directly beneath an overhead light source and then take one or two steps back. Now look directly into the mirror and see where the light naturally hits the face.

2, 3   Using downward strokes, apply bronzer with a fluffy brush to these light-hitting points. Start at the hairline and slowly build colour.

4, 5   Add a pinch of 'sunburn' by applying an orange/red cream to the fingertips and patting some lightly onto the cheeks.

contour made easy

A lot of people can make it feel like makeup is difficult and complicated. I'll let you in on a secret: it's not. It is, in fact, very easy. If it wasn't, then I certainly wouldn't be doing it! Once you understand the principles, which a lot of the time come down to placement, you can do anything. Take contouring, this is the placement of shadow in an area of the face or body to hollow it out. If you put that shadow in a different place, it becomes a blush. Let me share with you exactly where and how you should put your contour to win at shading every time.

Step by Step

1   First things first: placement. Using a large fluffy brush as a guide, place one end at the top of the ear and the other pointing to or touching the corner of the mouth.

2   Press the brush against the cheek to enable you to see where and in which direction the colour should go. Remove the brush and see if you can detect a slight mark where the brush pressed the skin, as this will help to guide you. Never assume: if you are unsure, then place the brush back to double check.

3   Find a colour, either cream or powder, that mimics the colour of the natural shadows found on your face (look under your chin or nose). Using the large fluffy brush, pick up a little of the colour on the tip of the brush only.

4   Starting at the back of the cheek bone (towards the top of the ear, as indicated with the brush earlier), sweep down in a straight line towards the corner of the mouth, without curving around the cheek. Let the brush flick off the skin for a softer gradient Repeat the brushstroke four or five times.

5   Brush over your application in the same angle and direction, slowly working towards the outer corner of the eye to wrap the contour around the cheek and soften the contour.

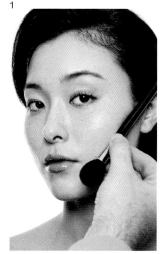
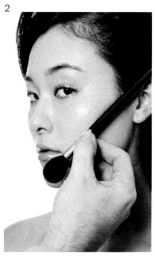
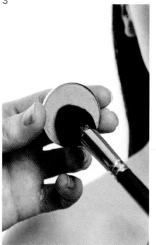
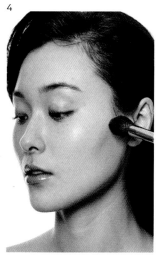
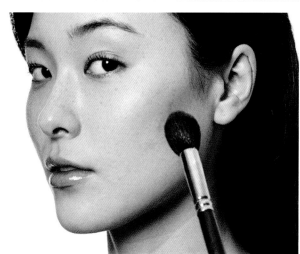

229

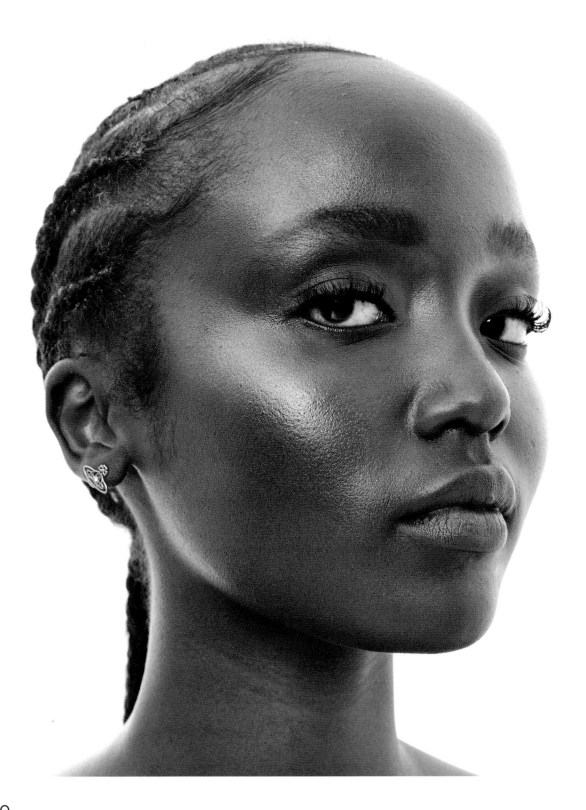

bold contour

One of the first things I was taught in makeup was a bronzing/contouring technique using the number three. Starting up on the temple, we would brush a large number three on the face, sweeping down onto the cheek and then back around and along the jawline. I always found this confusing, as it seemed odd that you would put a dark shade over the high point of the cheek that you actually want to keep bright and lifted. So I stopped doing the number three and started doing parallel lines instead. This technique not only intensifies the contour, but also enhances the highlighter, giving you a cheek that's as long as your arm and as sharp as a kitchen knife.

Step by Step

1   Using a large flat angled brush as a guide, place one end at the top of your ear and the other end pointing to or touching the corner of the mouth, as with the Contour Made Easy, p.229.

2   Keep the brush at the exact same angle, and move it up to the corner of the eye to show you the angle at which to apply a new contour up into the temple.

3   Apply the contour as on p.229, brushing down from the top of the ear to the corner of the mouth. Repeat this process from the temple to the corner of the eye.

4   Now take a large fluffy brush and sweep over the eyelid up towards the temple, over the outer edge of the brow and up into the hairline. Use the same brush to soften down the cheek contour.

5, 6   Take a highlighter, either cream or powder, and apply it with thumb and fingers above the brow arch and to the high point of the cheek to increase the contrast of the bone structure.

1
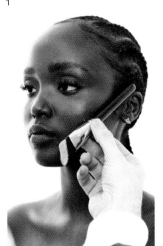

2
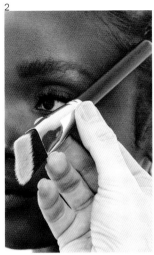

3
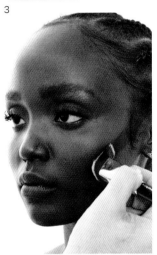

4
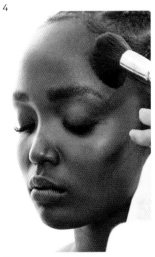

5
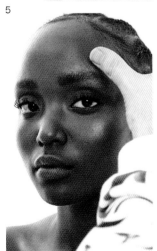

6
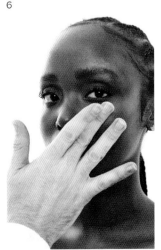

1
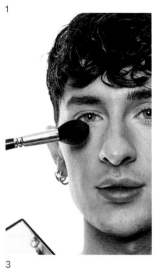

2
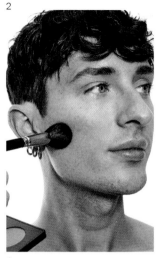

right angle contouring

Contour is intended to shape the face, and there are many ways to do this. It's all about adding a hollow or shadow to emphasise what is there. The angles we use can help to define the character of the contour. Using an angle that points down in a 45-degree slope can give the appearance of a slimmer or more elongated face shape. However, if you use angles that are more horizontal or vertical, these can give the appearance of a wider and stronger bone.

3
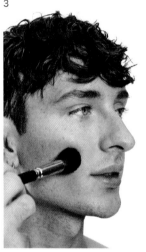

4
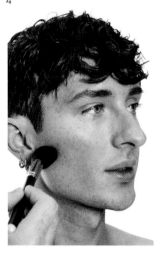

Step by Step

1   Using a medium fluffy brush, pick up some contour colour and place the brush directly under the iris then move it down in line with the bottom of the nose.

2   Sweep out and across towards the bottom of the ear in a straight line.

3   Go back to the original placement under the iris in line with the bottom of the nose and sweep straight down towards the ground.

4   Repeat steps 2 and 3 a couple of times until the edges are softened. Use a large fluffy brush to work over the contour to soften any edges, working towards the jawline.

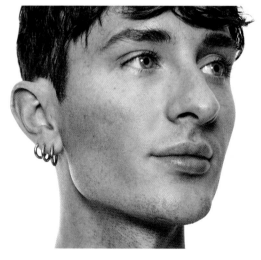

natural highlighter

For a natural looking highlighter, try reaching for a cream-based product. They melt into the skin to create a glow-from-within look rather than a frosted shimmer.

Step by Step

1 Looking at your bone structure in a mirror, identify the high points of your face; this is the area where light bounces off it.

2 Using your finger, position it on the part of the cheek directly under the outer corner of the eye. Apply a dot of cream/oil highlighter on this exact spot.

3 Tap your finger lightly either side of this point, moving down towards the apple of the cheek and up towards the top of the ear.

4 To really make your eyes pop, place a little of the highlighter above the arch of the brow, and blend up into the hairline above the temple.

5 Other areas to highlight could include the bridge of the nose and the cupid's bow.

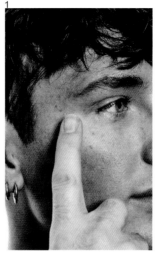
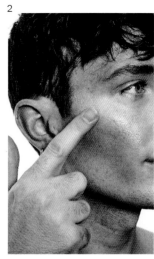
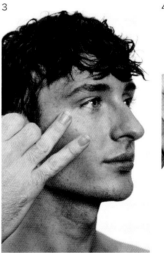
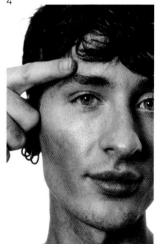
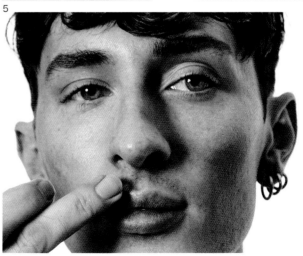

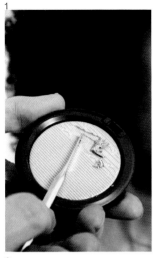

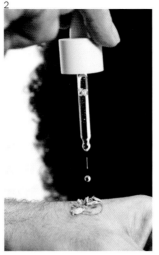

powder to liquid highlighter

I often get told by some people that powder highlighter doesn't work on them as it can enhance skin texture instead of smoothing it out. This can be true as highlighter reflects light but can also intensify shadow. One way to combat this is to use a liquid highlighter. If you don't have a liquid, use this hack to create your own and see how a liquid highlighter can make skin look smoother.

Step by Step

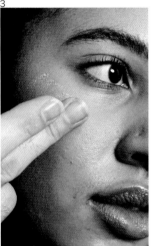

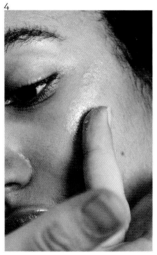

1,2   Scrape out some powder highlighter with a spatula or spoon. Tap this powder onto the back of your hand, or use a palette. Add a drop of facial oil and mix it all together with a finger or brush.

3–5   Apply this mixture to the high points on the face where the light would naturally hit, such as cheek bones, the bridge of the nose, cupid's bow and just above the arch of the brow.

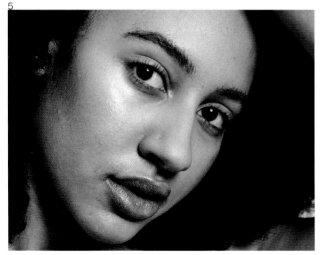

glitter highlighter

For a super intense highlighter, glitter can give a great high shine finish. But it doesn't need to be just for a festival or party. Use this technique to add a little extra pop to your everyday look to keep the party alive!

Step by Step

1   Apply cream highlighter along the cheekbones, around the temple and above the brow in an exaggerated 'C' shape.

2   Pour a small amount of different glitters into a tissue.

3   Form a pouch with the tissue by folding up the corners, and gently tap it to mix the glitters together.

4   Using a finger or fan brush, pick up the glitter and tap it onto the cheek, working up and around the 'C'.

5   Finish by applying a translucent glitter over your coloured glitter base for extra sparkle.

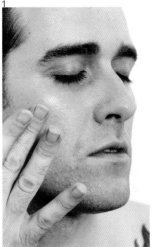
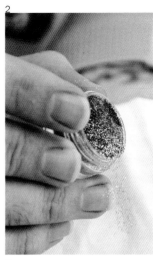
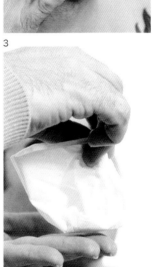
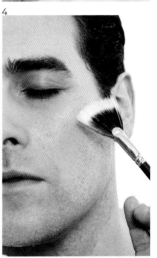
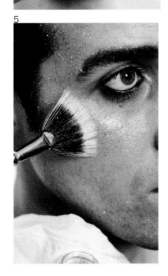
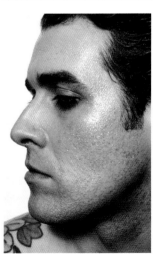

235

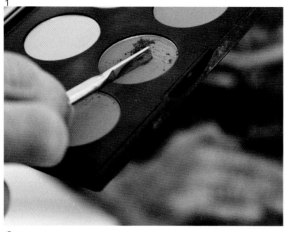

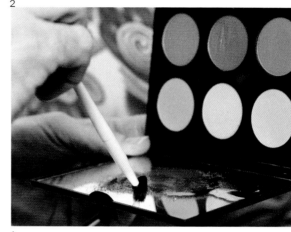

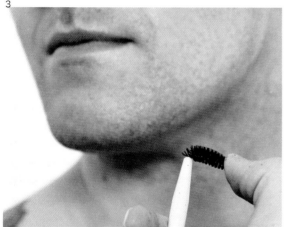

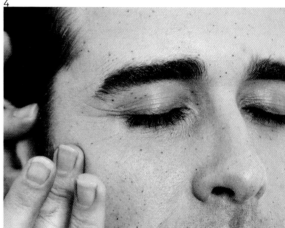

freckles made easy

Over the years, freckles have become a wonderful way to embrace one's individuality. What was once seen as something to cover is now something to highlight and enhance, or even create from scratch. To add a few freckles to your skin or increase the number you already have, try this super quick freckle hack.

Step by Step:

1   Scrape some dark pressed powder onto a mirror or a flat non-porous surface.

2   Use some water or makeup setting spray and mix this into the powder using a spoolie brush or clean toothbrush to create a muddy mixture.

3   Now flick towards your face using the spoolie brush.

4   Gently press your fingertip over the freckles to mute and soften some of them, being careful not to smear.

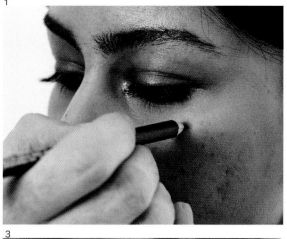

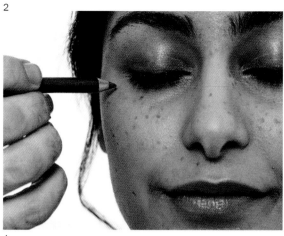

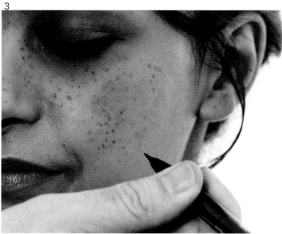

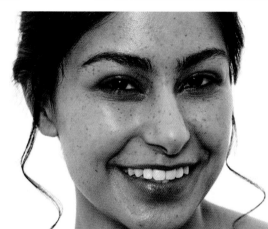

detailed freckles

The key to creating great freckles is to understand their nature. They are free spirited and random to the max in terms of placement, intensity and size. So for this technique, keep these three key words in mind.

Step by Step:

1   Select a few cool brown pencils, and start with the lightest shade. Press and twist the pencil onto the skin in small clusters to create groups of freckles. Use your fingertip to soften these dots into natural looking freckles.

2   Repeat this process with the medium and darker shades, making progressively fewer dots with the darkest shades.

3   Don't be afraid to add a few random, larger, darker and more prominent dots in places. Natural freckles are not uniform.

4   Repeat this process with a selection of felt brow-marker pens. Be sure to start with the lightest and apply the most dots with this shade, making fewer dots as you go darker.

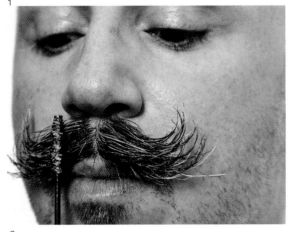
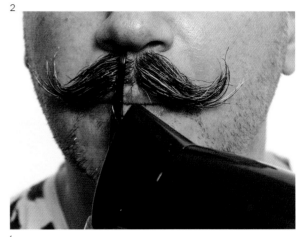
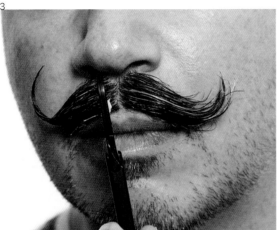
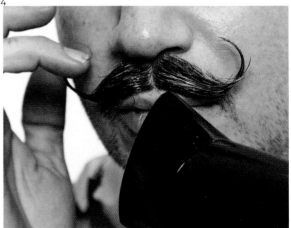

tash-tastic

Nothing suits everyone as much as a moustache! This fun-demental facial adornment adds style, uniqueness and personality to anyone who dare to wear it. I should know ;) All jokes aside, I get asked all the time how I style my 'tache so I felt it would be only appropriate to include my guide to facial hair finesse in this book. Don't knock it before you grow it!

Step by Step:

1   Take an eyebrow spoolie dipped in a super-strong hairstyling product and use it to brush the product through the moustache, starting under the moustache and brushing up. You can use any remaining product to brush brows up and out.

2   Using a moustache or lash and brow comb, blow dry the moustache out from the centre.

3   With a combe and then your fingers, pinch and twist the ends of the moustache into a curl.

4   Use the heat of the hairdryer to gently set the hair in place.

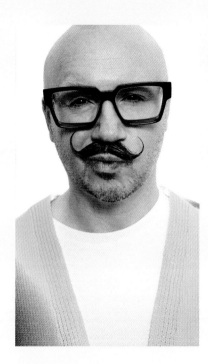

With thanks

The idea for this book was just that... an idea. I thought of what it could be if only I knew how. That is until a team of the most amazing individuals helped me bring it into reality. A huge thank you to Andrew Roff and Jennifer Barr for holding my hand through this process and keeping me to deadlines-ish. You made the process feel effortless and undaunting. Thank you to Renata Latipova for seeing the vision and steering the ship to the most beautiful inclusivity. You can not be what you can not see and in this book, everyone is seen. To Nikki Dupin, thank you for feeling the spirit of the book and designing something even better than what I saw in my head. Every page brings me so much joy and always something new to see. A huge thank you to Linda Shakesby for capturing the stunning images and all the fun, and sometimes chaos, on set. I know there were times when even I didn't know what was going to happen, but you somehow got it all so beautifully. Equally to Olivia Cartwright for having the constant supply of energy to keep everyone going, especially when we were starting to lose it a little. To my right hand, Wilma Stigson, your support both physically and mentally was enduring. You are insanely talented, and it was an honour to have you come along for the ride. A big thank you to Eddie Gold for believing in my vision and pulling out all the stops to make it happen. Also, to Izzy Toner for keeping a track of every step of this journey which was not easy when we didn't always know where we were going. Not forgetting the amazing models, thank you. You were all incredibly open to it all. You brought more than just your incredible faces, you brought you personality and your soul to each and every image. Finally, to my family, Thank You! Thank you for letting me get on with it. It can't have been easy at times to let me forge my own path even when I didn't know the destination, but your constant support and occasional picking up of pieces has led me to this place, where a Dyslexic kid with not much confidence can actually write a book. In a world where others might not understand you don't, for one second, consider yourself to be wrong.

Quarto

First published in 2024 by White Lion
an imprint of The Quarto Group.
One Triptych Place, London, SE1 9SH
United Kingdom
T (0)20 7700 6700
www.Quarto.com

A catalogue record for this book is available from the British Library.

ISBN 978-0-7112-9500-1
Ebook ISBN 978-0-7112-9501-8

Printed in China
10 9 8 7 6 5 4 3 2 1

Design and Art Direction Nikki Dupin for Studio Nic&lou

Publisher Jessica Axe
Commissioning Editor Andrew Roff
Editorial Director Jennifer Barr
Editorial Assistant Izzy Toner
Senior Designer Renata Latipova
Photography Assistant Olivia Cartwright
Additional Photography (moodboards) Louis Dupin
Hairstylist Wilma Stigson

Thank you to IMM Models, Zebedee Talent
and BAME Models for their talent.

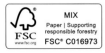